Covered

MY BREAST CANCER STORY & PRACTICAL INSIGHT FOR YOURS

TANYA MOTORIN

COVERED
My Breast Cancer Story and Practical Insight for Yours
Copyright © 2023 by Tanya Motorin

All scriptures, unless otherwise noted, were taken from the Holy Bible, New International Version®, NIV®. Copyright © 1973, 1978, 1984, 2011 by Biblica, Inc.™ Used by permission of Zondervan. All rights reserved worldwide. www.zondervan.com The "NIV" and "New International Version" are trademarks registered in the United States Patent and Trademark Office by Biblica, Inc.™

Any internet addresses (websites, blogs, etc.) and telephone numbers in this book are offered as a resource. They are not intended in any way to be or imply an endorsement by The Unknown Authors Club, nor does The Unknown Authors Club vouch for the content of these sites and numbers for the life of this book.

All rights reserved. No part of this publication may be reproduced, stored in a retrieval system, or transmitted in any form or by any means—electronic, mechanical, photocopy, recording, or any other—except for brief quotations in printed reviews, without the prior permission of the publisher.

Requests for information should be addressed to:
The Unknown Authors Club
P.O. Box 170397
Boise, Idaho 83717
www.theunknownauthorsclub.com

Softcover ISBN: 979-8-9868277-4-2
eBook ISBN: 979-8-9868277-5-9

Cover design: Leslee Stewart
Interior design: Rachel Langaker

Printed in the United States of America.

To Nikita, Hope, Sophia and Zion. As I walked this deep and unfamiliar valley, your presence brought peace to quiet my fears, strength I was lacking, and the hope I so desperately needed to hold on to. There are no words to describe my love for you.

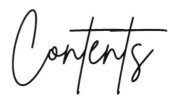

Contents

Foreword by Joy Eggerichs Reed	9
Preface: From Me to You	15

MY STORY

1. Letter to Cancer	23
2. The Day the Wheels Came Off	27
3. Best.Birthday.Ever	33
4. Now What?	37
5. Goodbye Emerald City	41
6. Telling The Kids	45
7. Why Suffering?	55
8. A Different Kind of Love	65

YOUR STORY
ESSENTIALS FOR THE JOURNEY

9. Find Your A-Team	79
10. Making Space for Grief	91

11. Permission	101
12. Be Kind to Yourself	117
13. Celebrate Along the Way	123

GETTING DOWN TO BUSINESS

14. Breast Surgeon: Surgery Decisions	133
15. Plastic Surgeon: Reconstruction Decisions	137
16. Genetic Testing	141
17. Stepping into Battle	145

NECESSARY EVILS & DISAPPOINTING NEWS

18. Waiting for Results	153
19. Incidental Findings	157
20. Oncology	161
21. Chemo	169
22. Radiation	179

HAIR & BEAUTY

23: Hair 101	187
24: Hair After Treatment	207
25: The Beauty Bar	215

LIFE AFTER CANCER

26. Back from War	225
27. Pursuing Wellness	231
28. Sex and Intimacy	247
29. Silver Linings	255
30. Kintsugi: Golden Repair	261
31. Insight for Those Beside You	267
To My Hall-Of-Famers	299
Notes	307
About The Author	311

Foreword

BY JOY EGGERICHS REED

I was walking around in the shallow end of a pool in Santa Barbara, California soaking in the Mediterranean climate where I enjoyed four spoiled years of college. My parents had flown out to be with me after recently graduating and I am confident that as Michigan residents, they were happy to be soaking in the sun as well. I now enjoyed being with my parents and was finally through the flippant teenage stage where I wanted distance from them. The infamous day in high school where I yelled, "Just face it dad, mom, and I will NEVER be friends!" was becoming a story we could now laugh about.

I remember my mom was in the pool with me and my dad was sitting on the edge. I don't remember exactly how it came out, but they told me that they wanted to tell me something in person. They then proceeded to share that my mom had been diagnosed with breast cancer. Had it not been for the cradling magic of the water, I'm sure my knees would have buckled, dropping me to the ground.

A million questions raced through my brain, including the selfish ones like, "Will she be at my wedding or around to help if I have kids?" Then of course the shame of thinking through all the years I wasted being in my own world at college and probably only calling or emailing when I needed something. Because in my mind, CANCER equaled DEATH and this was the end.

Once I could finally hear my parents through my own extreme thoughts, I realized they had an action plan. My parents are very comfortable with talking about the inevitability of death and suffering and that both of those things are something none of us can escape in this life. After they gave their theology lessons, they also shared the news that this was something the doctors believed could be cured for now. There were many large pendulum swings of emotions, sermons and dark daydreams in that shallow end of the pool that day.

So, I changed my plans for the following year and traded Mediterranean for the Midwest and took care of my mother after her double mastectomy. I remember emptying tubes of fluid and being affirmed that a medical nurse was probably not my calling. I remember being proud of my mom, who usually moves at the pace of a rabbit on speed and finally slowed down to watch a movie with me. She couldn't really move much so she finally had to get a taste of *my* favorite activity which is being a couch potato and moving at the pace of a sedated snail.

My mother was 52 at the time and we are now almost twenty years removed from that destabilizing day in the pool and her forced film binging. She is over seventy years old and can run circles around me. And even though I didn't get married and start a family until my mid-thirties, my initial selfish thoughts of, "...but I need her to be at my wedding and help raise my kids," were all realized.

I know that's not the case for everyone. Some battles drag on for years, relapses happen, and loved ones are lost before babies are born or diplomas at graduations are given. It's all too much.

Tanya Motorin knows the "too much" first hand.

When I learned about Tanya's book and her hope to help those who have been diagnosed with breast cancer as well as their caretakers, I wanted to immediately see the table of contents. Not only is this book a story of another young, healthy woman getting her world altered and feminine identity shaken, but it is also extremely practical.

It was a bittersweet season for me when I took care of my mom. I am so thankful I had that time to spend with her, but I also felt ill-equipped and out of my depth. My dad was doing all the research and talking to the doctors, but now seeing Tanya's book, I know I would have devoured a resource like this as well as my mom.

I'm sure I wasn't thinking about what type of food to feed my mom and I don't even think the genetic testing was available when she was diagnosed. And I also wasn't thinking about intimate details of how this was impacting my mother as a woman.

So much of cancer is sterile and medical, as it needs to be, but it's also a deep dive into the human psyche. For the patient and caretakers, the word "unprepared" feels so fitting because, *who prepares for cancer*??

A cancer diagnosis is like learning you have a college exam tomorrow and you now have to pull an all-nighter cramming to become an expert and hopefully pass a test you didn't know existed three hours ago. Of course you have the "library" of doctor's advice and information but that can be daunting and conflicting.

Tanya is here to greet you and your loved ones at that library door, walk you to the one random cozy area near the periodicals that traded out fiberglass chairs from the 50s for a few couches and some coffee tables.

She will sit you down, hand you a cup of coffee and say, "We are gonna pull this all-nighter together. You are not alone, I have already studied for the test and kept my notes. I pulled from the resources that will help you pass and put them together for you here in this book. I even encourage you to journal, reflect, and make this study time your own, but more than anything I don't want you to add any more stress to your life than you already have just encountered by the sheer surprise of learning about the upcoming exam."

She pours you a second cup of coffee and will be available during this long night whenever you need her.

Thank you Tanya for taking the time to hold the hand of so many. I wish you would have been at my library twenty years ago, but I'm thankful you're making yourself available now.

Joy Eggerichs Reed
author of *Get to the Publishing Punchline*

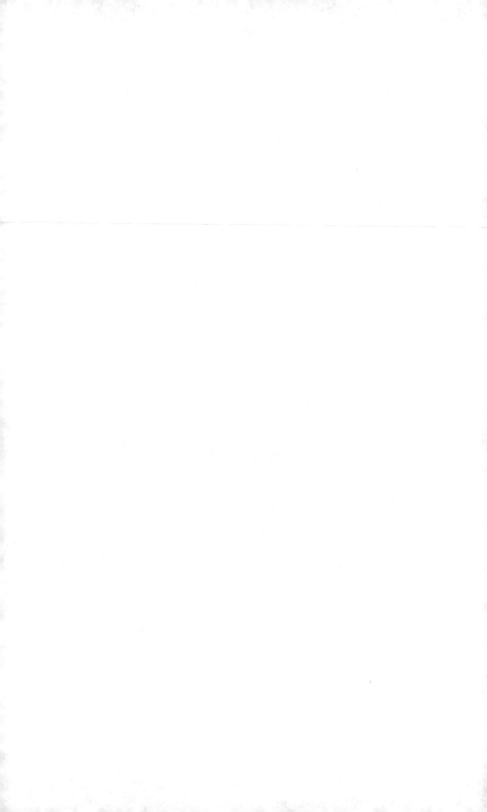

Preface

FROM ME TO YOU

I know. I hate it too. I hate that this book is in your hands. I hate that I had to write it. I hate that breast cancer is part of my story, and I hate that it's part of yours now too. I never wanted to be in a place where the word "cancer" was used in the same sentence with my name; I know you can relate. Sometimes I still shake my head and wonder how this ugly word came into my world. It's awful and life-altering. It's scary and overwhelming beyond words. It's unknown and isolating. I know.

I'm not saying that I can understand exactly what you are going through, because no breast cancer diagnosis is exactly the same, but I can relate to the ups and downs of a breast cancer diagnosis, and I know that this path you are on can feel disorienting and devastating. I want you to know that I'm with you, and I want you to know that this book is for you. You are the reason I was compelled to get my words on paper.

I always wanted to write a book, but I never knew what I wanted to write about. I thought maybe a children's book or a topical book, but I wasn't sure that I had enough to say about any one topic. As soon as I got my diagnosis, I thought, *Well, I guess I know what I'm writing my book about!* I didn't choose the topic—it chose me. Even though I share my story with you in these pages, this book isn't just a cathartic way for me to process all that I've been through (although it has been that); this book is for you, too. As you read, I want this book to be a place that you can run to when you feel like no one else really gets it. I want you to know that you are not alone. No matter how much your friends and family love you and are surrounding you, it's not the same as talking to someone who has walked this path before you. A breast cancer diagnosis shatters your world, and I am heartbroken that you too, are having to go through this.

My hope is that this book will be a lifeline for you when you feel like you are drowning. A place that brings a bit of peace and clarity, or just retreat, as you navigate through the overwhelming world of tests, diagnosis, surgery, and treatment, not to mention the array of emotions that come along with all of those things, like some kind of "buy one get one free" deal. On a given day, you might experience fear, confusion, despair, anger, hopelessness, and a myriad of other "fun" emotions. It's a lot to carry and sort through. I hope that our time together will feel like pulling up a chair with a friend who understands, and a nurse-navigator that can help walk you through the practical elements that are completely overwhelming.

This is the book I wish I would have had when I was battling cancer.

In these pages, you'll read my story, from the moment I heard the word "cancer," to where I am now. Threaded throughout is practical advice I learned along the way. Some of it is advice others shared with me, but I also include lessons I had to learn the hard way—like when I ended up with a wig that wasn't what I needed because I didn't know what to look for, or when I learned to be kind to myself when I wasn't "mom and wife of the year" during my cancer treatment.

After I was diagnosed, I immediately reached out to anyone and everyone I knew who had faced breast cancer. I never felt like I had enough time to ask all my questions, but when those old and new friends shared with me, I would take notes as fast as I could. I didn't want to miss any of their wisdom because I had no clue what I was heading into. Just like those who took me by the hand, I've also had the privilege of helping others who have been diagnosed after me. Along the way, I began to wonder if there was a better way to pass along my knowledge and experience.

So, even though I wish we could sit down face to face and share our stories, this book is my way to share my journey and pass along my best practices and advice to you. My hope is that the words on these pages minister to you and help lighten the load.

Keep in mind, I'm not a doctor or researcher, so my advice is not medically proven; I simply offer what has worked (or not worked) for me, in hopes that my advice might be helpful for you. At the end of the book, I also include tips and insight on how those around you can care for you during this time. If your "people" are anything like my "people," they will want to help, but they may need some guidance. Hopefully, this section will help them, and ultimately you.

As you read, you will also encounter a number of blog posts from my CaringBridge website. CaringBridge is a website that provides a free online space for people facing health challenges to stay connected with those around them. I wanted to include some of my CaringBridge posts to give you a real-time glimpse into my world as I navigated the heartbreak and victories that come with a cancer diagnosis.

If you have been newly diagnosed and you are in need of immediate direction and practical first steps to take, I would recommend skipping straight to the section entitled, "Essentials for the Journey." Here you will find helpful information you will need from the very beginning of your journey with breast cancer. Once you've read through this section, you can go back to read my story or feel free to skim the table of contents to find a section that pertains to what you are currently wading through.

I also thought I should share a quick disclaimer before you start reading. Much of what I share with you will have a faith influence, because of my background. As you read my story, you'll learn about my battle with cancer, as well as my internal wrestling with fear and trying to trust a God who allows this kind of suffering. I thought about leaving the faith element out, because I know it's not for everyone, but it's so intertwined into who I am and what I've been through, I found it impossible to write my story without also sharing my struggles and breakthroughs with God along the way. I wish that God had chosen a different way to teach me, mature me, and draw me near to Him, but cancer was the "teacher" He chose for me. I hope instead of pushing you away, sharing my faith perspective will care for your heart and soul, because this isn't just a physical battle, but a spiritual and emotional one as well. However, I don't want the spiritual thread woven throughout this book to keep you from getting the practical help you may need. Even if you and God aren't exactly simpatico, I'm wondering if this might be the time when you need Him more than ever. I think C.S. Lewis might have been onto something when he wrote, "Pain is God's megaphone."[1] I know this has been true for me.

Maybe you've picked up this book and your faith background is similar to mine. You consider yourself a Christ-follower, and you want to continue trusting Him through this deep and dark valley, but your faith is feeling a bit shaky. It may be hard to know if you can trust God when He allows this kind of pain to reach you. There's something in here for you as well. I invite you to journey with me through my victories and devastation and, perhaps as we walk together, something will resonate with you and help you to see God's heart more clearly. I hope so.

On many days through this journey, I found myself grasping for words that could match the chaos and heartbreak wreaking havoc on me, and I just came up empty handed. I would either sit in silence with my shoulders shaking and tears streaming down my face, or I would wait until everyone had left the house and I would curse at the top of my lungs. I know it's not in the prayer handbook for what I'm "supposed" to pray, but when you are raw and broken, you don't have the strength to filter your prayers. God had to just deal with the unedited version of me, and if I'm totally honest, I think that's the version He prefers. I hope that my authenticity will also give you permission to come to God just as you are.

Wherever you stand with God, you are welcome here. I wish we could have met under different circumstances, but I'm thankful for the courage you have shown by opening up this book. You have been unwillingly initiated into this breast cancer club and I know that it must feel like one of the darkest and scariest times in your life. I wish that I could rewrite your story—and mine. Since I can't, my prayer is that you will find some peace in knowing that you are not alone.

Standing with you,

PART 1

My Story

GOD IS OUR REFUGE AND STRENGTH, AN EVER-PRESENT HELP IN TROUBLE. THEREFORE WE WILL NOT FEAR, THOUGH THE EARTH GIVE WAY AND THE MOUNTAINS FALL INTO THE HEART OF THE SEA, THOUGH ITS WATERS ROAR AND FOAM AND THE MOUNTAINS QUAKE WITH THEIR SURGING. THERE IS A RIVER WHOSE STREAMS MAKE GLAD THE CITY OF GOD, THE HOLY PLACE WHERE THE MOST HIGH DWELLS. GOD IS WITHIN HER, SHE WILL NOT FALL; GOD WILL HELP HER AT BREAK OF DAY.

PSALM 46:1-5 NIV

Chapter 1

LETTER TO CANCER

April 4, 2019

cancer.

What a horrible word. I'm not capitalizing you because you don't deserve honor and I'm not writing "dear" before you because you aren't dear. You are the opposite of dear. What would that be?

Crappy? Stupid? Ridiculous? Messed up?

How dare you. You don't even deserve my words, but since Karrie, my therapist, asked me to write you a letter, I'm doing it. Because that's who I am. I try to be faithful to God and others. I want to be obedient. I always try to follow through. I try to be someone who will breathe life into others, so that they will be changed for the better after spending time with me. In fact, I decided to spend the last eighteen years of my life serving God because my heart breaks for people who don't know Him.

In fact, I think it's ironic that countless times I have shared with athletes and others who don't know Jesus, that the sin and selfishness in our lives is like a cancer, a cancer that is causing brokenness in our hearts and destroying us and those around us. Then I would go on to ask them, *What if I had the cure to cancer and I could heal so many people, but I chose not to share it. Or just kept it to myself. What?!? Who would do that? Not me, I would share it with everyone.* Now more than any other time, that analogy takes on new meaning for me.

You barged your way into my life. Uninvited. Not welcome. How dare you. I thought for sure that I had too many other details to worry about with packing up our home, moving, saying goodbye to life in Seattle, driving to CA, finding a place to live, and a school for our kids. Surely, I would get a free pass this time. Right?

Wrong. How dare you come into my body. My breast. The breast that nourished my kids and brought them life. The breast that brought my husband so much pleasure. How dare you.

When I first heard your name in the ultrasound room, I wanted to hit rewind. I couldn't believe that you and I were in the same room. You. The one who took my grandma. My aunt. My friends. The one who threatened to take my mom. How dare you show up the day before my 46th birthday and start pushing me around like a bully. How dare you threaten me, and infuse me with fear. How dare you take my lunch and feed me lies instead. How dare you begin to chip away at my foundation and bring quakes that shook me to the core. Quakes that made me question the One who has always been been my steady foundation.

I looked at you and wondered why. Why me? Why now? Why would God allow this? I was filled with fear. You showed up on the scene and you were an ugly skyscraper blocking my view of the beautiful snowcapped mountains. You overshadowed everything. My days were filled with fear, and grief, and so many tears. You were depleting me.

Hitting me when I turned around. Hitting me below the belt. You weren't playing by the rules and suddenly I felt pinned by you. How dare you.

BUT, you don't get the final word. Just because you barged in and stood taller (for a time) than everything else in my life, one day the sun poked out from behind the clouds and I realized that the beautiful mountains were still there. I just needed to walk around this monstrous skyscraper and look up. They were still there. He was still there. He had never left me and He wasn't forsaking me, just like He had promised before I ever met Him. Even though the landscape of my "city" had changed, His presence and His beauty wasn't going away. I just needed to change my perspective.

So guess what? Your boss (yes, I know who sent you) didn't win. He's already been defeated, so long ago by my Creator. Even though you seem scary when you are towering over me, when I step out of your shadow I feel His warmth and goodness again. He is victorious, therefore, I am victorious! What you meant for evil, God meant for good.

Your boss has only come to steal, kill, and destroy, but my Father has come that I might have life. Life to the full. So I'm claiming this abundant life that He has promised. Guess what that means? Game over. You're a joke. How dare you think that you could defeat me and my God.

Go home loser.

Tanya

Chapter 2

THE DAY THE WHEELS CAME OFF

Our family called Seattle home for six years. It was in Seattle I learned that I don't actually love the rain as much as I thought, where my husband became a coffee snob, and where we bought our first house. My dad had died a couple of years into our time in Seattle, and after such a deep loss, I had been feeling the tug to move back to Southern California where I had grown up in order to be closer to my mom and the rest of my family. With Nikita, my husband, being from Kazakhstan and me being from California, I often wondered why in the world we were both living so far from our families. It made sense on paper to move closer to one of our families, but it just wasn't that simple since we had spent six years writing a significant chapter of our family's life in the Pacific Northwest.

Though it was difficult to think of replanting our family again, in the Spring of 2018, we began the completely overwhelming process of sorting through our things, taking a million trips to the Goodwill, packing, checking off our Seattle bucket list, supporting our local Target by finding their cheapest, stylish home decor items to stage our house, soaking up time with our friends, and listing the first home we had ever owned on the market. It was exhausting and heart-wrenching. Every day, I wanted to cry and sleep—but there was just too much that had to be done, and I desperately wanted to finish well in Seattle.

In the midst of all of our preparations to move to LA, I was also busy trying to fit in dental appointments and annual doctor visits for our family so we didn't have to deal with all of that while we were settling in.

I was grinding and daily checking things off my "to do" list until I got a call that stopped me in my tracks. It was a follow-up call from Seattle Breast Imaging saying that after my routine mammogram a couple of days before, they needed more images. Since I had just gotten a "normal" breast exam the day before at my annual OBGYN appointment, I reassured myself that they probably just needed clearer images and that would be it. I was also counting on the fact that between packing boxes and trying to squeeze every ounce out of Seattle, I figured that God knew that I literally could not handle a curveball.

Apparently, the mammogram technician didn't get that memo though, because when I went back for more images, she pulled and yanked my boob in every direction imaginable, and when it was smushed as flat as a Parisian crepe, they found a concerning spot and decided to do an ultrasound that day.

Back to the waiting room I went. I remember just staring straight ahead and trying to pray. I texted my husband who was wondering why I had been gone for so long and simply wrote, "It's not good." All I wanted was to have him next to me, holding my hand tight. Instead, I felt alone, yet I was surrounded by other anxious women waiting and wondering how this could be happening. To pass time, I prayed for each woman who came through the door as I wondered what they were thinking and feeling, and whether or not they were about to be blindsided as well.

The nurse brought me back to a room to wait some more. When the radiologist finally came in, she showed me my mammogram images and pointed out one concerning area, and then she matter of factly told me she was pretty certain it was cancer. *Wait.* What did she just say?

No. This was not happening. *No, no, no.* I mean, after nursing three kids and then finally losing the baby weight, I barely had any boobs to fill up my padded bra—how could there even be cancer in there? She had to be wrong, or I had to be dreaming. I wanted to either throw up or wake up. I barely had time to fit this appointment in, how could I possibly find time to deal with a life-threatening diagnosis? I wanted my old problems back. *Noooo.* Couldn't I just go back to complaining about the weather and how isolated I felt in Seattle? How was it possible that one day I was emotionally and physically spent, but excited about our next chapter in California, and the next day I found myself in the middle of an absolute nightmare? *Un-freakin-believable.* I wondered if God knew I already felt as though I was sinking.

As the radiologist started the ultrasound, she found a couple more spots in my breast, and when I told her I was moving that Sunday (six days later), she stopped the ultrasound and asked if I was okay with her stepping out for a minute to ask the other doctor if he would fit me in to biopsy the most concerning spot that day. She came back a few minutes later to confirm that the doctor could do the biopsy. She finished up the ultrasound as I stared ahead in silence. My head was spinning with fear and panic. I had a million questions, and yet I had lost my words. A few minutes later, a doctor without a personality or an ounce of empathy came in to do the biopsy, and then they sent me on my way.

As I drove home that day with a bandage on my breast, I felt as if someone had just mugged me and then enlisted me for war, without my consent. Surprisingly, there were no tears. Not yet. I was in complete shock and drove on autopilot as I navigated the traffic on Montlake Avenue. As I made my way home, I felt God was reassuring me, "You're not the first or the last woman to go through this. But I AM the first and the last. The beginning and the end." I had no idea what I was really walking into, but He did, and He reminded me that He was with me before the wheels fell off, and He would be with me long after.

Chapter 3

BEST.BIRTHDAY.EVER.

The next day was my 46th birthday. Yay for me. I normally LOVE celebrating birthdays, mine and others, but for this birthday, all I really wanted to do was curl up in a ball by myself and cry until there were no tears left. Instead, I tapped into my acting skills from my high school theater days, and I completely faked it as our family went to CJ's, our favorite Seattle breakfast spot to "celebrate." Nikita and I wanted to keep things as normal as possible in the midst of the chaos we were already living, so the kids had no idea what was going on. After breakfast, we walked through Pike Place Market (where everyone goes when they want to be alone), wandered along the waterfront, and then we headed home to resume packing.

A few hours later, I got the call. I motioned for Nikita to come into the bedroom with me and we held our breath as we waited for what felt like days before hearing the words, "Invasive Ductal Carcinoma." It was like a foreign language, but I knew it meant cancer. Nikita and I stayed in our room after I hung up. I just stared at him as my eyes filled with tears. He reached out his hand and then held me as I silently wept. *How was this happening?* I wondered. *Happy birthday to me, happy birthday to me, happy birthday dear Tanya, happy birthday to me.* Best. Birthday. Ever.

Before I got the call, I think I was still holding out hope that there was some kind of mistake. Maybe there was still a chance my life wasn't disintegrating in front of my eyes. As I tried to catch my breath, there was no denying my reality. This was really happening.

Though I had so many questions, one thing crystalized: I had felt compelled by God to move closer to my family years before, and now I knew why. They would be standing with me and keeping me steady when things became blurry on the road ahead. God was graciously preparing a place of safety and care for me to fight this battle. Everything else would be built around this anchor.

Все будет хорошо (Everything's Gonna Be Okay)

CaringBridge Journal Entry by Tanya Motorin
October 31, 2018

When I lived in Kazakhstan, the locals there had a saying that completely drove me nuts. Whenever you were frustrated or worried about something, they would listen to you share and then nine times out of ten they would respond by saying, "Все будет хорошо." They must have taught them this phrase in the Soviet schools because everyone knew it, and everyone used it. All. The. Time.

Translated into English, it means, "Everything's gonna be okay." It sounds like a harmless thing to say, but I couldn't stand it when people would say this to me because it just seemed like they were trying to put a Band-aid on a wound that required surgery. And on top of that, how did they know that everything was going to be okay?

It's ironic to me that from the first day that I received this diagnosis and Nikita just held me as the news began to sink in, the first thing I asked him to say to me was, "Все будет хорошо." I didn't know how it would be okay, but I wanted to be reassured that everything was going to be okay. That our family was going to be okay. That I was going to be okay. I just needed to hear those words.

Now that I am three months in, I still don't like the path I'm on, but I am thankful to be learning more about the companion I'm on this journey with. As I read Psalm 29 yesterday, I was reminded that He doesn't always take us out of our difficult situations, but we don't have to face them alone. Verses 10-11[1] say this:

The Lord sits enthroned over the flood;
the Lord is enthroned as King forever.
The Lord gives strength to his people;
the Lord blesses his people with peace.

Even though I don't know how everything will be okay, I have to trust that He is the King enthroned over the flood in my life. When the waters are rushing and strong, and I think I might be carried away by the flood's power, I look up and see my King in power OVER the flood. Not only is He in power, He gives me what I need. The last thing I can muster up right now is strength and peace, so I am so very thankful that God knows what I need even before I ask for it. And yesterday what I needed was this reminder that He is still King, and because of that, everything's gonna be okay.

Chapter 4

NOW WHAT?

After getting the news, I wanted to crumble, but there was no time for that (yet), I had to get crap done. The next day, I reached out to our good friend Dennis Woo, who was a pediatrician at UCLA and whose wife had also battled breast cancer years before. As we talked, he was the perfect blend of compassion, love, empathy, and let's get down to business. He encouraged me to reread the book of Job in the Bible, like he and his wife had done in the midst of her diagnosis. What stuck with me during that conversation is what Job said to his wife when she was telling him to curse God and die, "You talk like a foolish woman. Should we accept only good things from the hand of God and never anything bad?"[1] I wanted to shout, "Yes! Good things, only good things." But I knew that wasn't how life worked. I couldn't be the only one immune from pain and suffering. And if I was going to become like Him, who had also experienced pain and suffering, I would also have to walk through it. It sounded logical on paper, but in the middle of my suffering, I wanted to dig my heals in and keep myself from experiencing this kind of heartache. At the very same time, my head was telling me I had to accept my new reality.

I asked Dennis who I should contact, and he got me in touch with Dr. Helena Chang, a breast surgeon at UCLA. I later discovered she was the Director of the Revlon Breast Center at UCLA. Once again, I saw that God wasn't choosing to pull me out of the pain and suffering, but instead, He wanted me to see His perfect provision in the midst of it.

The soonest I could get in to see Dr. Chang was three weeks later, which felt like an eternity when you have cancer in your body, but in between packing boxes and staging our home, I didn't have the time or headspace to research and call different doctors. I had to trust that God was providing for me through Dennis, so I took the appointment and tried to not be completely paralyzed while I waited.

There would be so many more decisions to be made, but for now, I had the first one in place. This was the last path I wanted to walk down, but if I had to go through this, it was reassuring knowing that when I rolled in to LA, there would be a breast surgeon waiting for me.

Chapter 5

GOODBYE EMERALD CITY

The next day the movers came and I started my period. Moving, exhaustion, a one day-old cancer diagnosis, cramps, and hormones. The perfect storm.

As reality sank in that we were leaving our home of six years, and I had cancer currently in my body, I needed space to cry and scream, or hit something. I wanted so desperately to be alone and throw a tantrum. But I wasn't going to get any of this. Long before the word cancer invaded our story, we had promised the kids that we could camp out a couple of nights in the backyard before we started our drive to California. Of course at this point I was wondering why in the world I had agreed to this. But there was no backing out. Once we promise something to our kids, they are like bloodhounds until they get it. And besides, we couldn't use the cancer card because Nikita and I still hadn't told them anything. We wanted to wait until we knew more and the kids had some time to settle into the new rhythms of life in LA.

So, what did we do? We pitched our tent and stayed for a couple more days. We went to all our favorite spots one more time, but I was just going through the motions. On the outside I was doing my best to finish well, but on the inside, I was a basket case. Despite my best efforts, the bitter was overpowering the sweet and I felt as though I was covered by the darkest, most threatening cloud covering I'd ever seen in that rainy city.

The time finally came for us to pack up the tent and the last of our belongings. In some ways I wanted to stay forever and try to salvage the "normal" life I used to have. After all, this was where we had brought home our son from the hospital and where our girls had spent the majority of their lives. We had hosted countless dinners, game nights, Bible studies, bridal showers, premarital counseling, birthday parties, family Thanksgiving, and out-of-town guests. And Nikita had renovated nearly every room in our 1927 home. But sadly, that normal life no longer existed.

I was so scared to walk forward and learn what this diagnosis really meant. Since running away or hiding wasn't an option, I had to keep walking on the path that God had for me and my family. This wasn't how I envisioned our return to California, but I couldn't deny the fact that He was calling us back home.

My eyes were filled with tears as I took one more look inside our home and then slowly closed our front door for the last time. We took a family selfie in front of our sweet home, piled in the car, said a quick prayer, and headed south. As I looked out the window, I watched our old life slip away and wondered what lay ahead of us in the Golden State.

Instead of enjoying the scenery on a long road trip, I was texting my friends to tell them about my diagnosis and quietly crying, watching the miles tick by. I wished I had space to call my friends and openly grieve with them. Instead, as I texted each of them, I asked them to pray, but I told them not to call me during our drive so the kids wouldn't get suspicious. I'm not sure how I was functioning, but despite our emotional and physical exhaustion, we made it to my mom's in Southern California. After the kids went down for bed, my mom and I cried, hugged, shook our heads, and wondered together, *How is this happening?*

Chapter 6
TELLING THE KIDS

When Nikita and I decided not to tell the kids right away, it wasn't because we were trying to shelter them or pretend like everything was fine, but because of the major life turmoil they were already experiencing. We had just uprooted them and started over in the City of Angels, then two weeks later, they started school. We were all getting our footing in our new world, so telling them I had cancer just didn't seem like the thing they needed in the midst of so much change and uncertainty. I'll admit that there was part of me that wanted to find every excuse possible not to tell them, ever. I couldn't bear the thought of seeing the fear and confusion in their eyes. Usually when something difficult happens to us, we don't know it's coming, but I knew that I had really scary news for them. It felt horrible that they had no idea what was about to hit them. I needed to get the move behind us and get them situated in school and then we would do the next hard thing.

Since we had never been through cancer before, we had to make a game time decision and we decided to wait. I know that everyone handles situations like this differently, but for me, I know my kids, and I knew that we needed to wait. After all, being uprooted, leaving the city in which they had spent the majority of their lives, saying goodbye to their friends and heading to a new city with new everything…it was just too much. Fear on top of a bunch of sadness, doesn't make for a great recipe. Plus, if we did tell them, I knew they would have asked me every single question in the book, and I didn't have any answers for them. I'm confident that telling them immediately would have brought more harm than help. That was the last thing I wanted for them as they were already being stretched far beyond comfortable.

So, we made the decision to wait, but this led to a different obstacle I hadn't thought through. Now instead of wearing my heart on my sleeve like I normally do, I had to pretend as though I was my normal self. It was torture. They saw me crying a lot, but I think they assumed that I was sad about leaving Seattle. Even now as I think back to those days, I shudder. It really was hell and I was trying my hardest to keep them away from the flames for as long as possible.

We moved into our rental on a Saturday and the kids started school the following Tuesday. We snapped a first day of school photo with their new outfits and their bravest faces. Other than Kindergarten, I never had to start at a new school not knowing a soul. My heart was breaking for them and yet, I was bursting with pride at the same time. Could it be that God was using this new experience to build their faith and resiliency muscles to prepare them for what lay ahead? I know that God doesn't waste anything, so I trusted that there were lessons being learned that would strengthen them for the next chapter.

They got through their first week, and even though they didn't want to stay after school to play like they used to in Seattle, they each had made connections with sweet kids and had even been invited on playdates. My mama's heart was so relieved. They were going to be okay. They weren't going to hate us forever for uprooting them, and before we knew it, they were going to be thriving again.

Now that their first week was behind them, I knew that we needed to tell them, but I wanted to wait a little bit longer. I don't know if it was God, or if I was just putting off a really hard conversation, but everything in me wanted to protect them from more hard stuff. I wanted to let them be kids for a little longer. When I was a kid, the hardest things I dealt with were when my mom bought chicken hot dogs instead of beef, or when my neighbor pulled down my tube top in front of the other neighborhood kids. Granted, it's no fun for a 9-year-old to be humiliated in front of her peers, but it wasn't cancer. I wanted to keep my kids' world as carefree and beautiful for as long as possible.

By this point, I had met with my new doctor in LA and had a surgery date—September 26th. Now it was official. It wasn't something out there that may or may not happen. This next chapter was beginning whether I was ready or not and I knew it was time. I needed to honor my children's need for time and space to process and prepare their hearts for the storm heading their way.

I had no idea how to even start the conversation. I was thankful that the kids were used to having our regular family meetings when we could all check in, work through conflict with one another, share highs and lows, and talk about family news and upcoming events. About a month before my surgery, we told the kids we wanted to have a family meeting. Thankfully they didn't see our request as anything new or unusual.

Nikita and I had decided ahead of time that I would be the one to tell them and he would fill in the gaps. He had offered to lead the conversation, but I felt like they needed to hear it from me. After doing our "check in" time, I told them I had something I needed to share with them. It went something like this...

Do you guys remember when we were getting ready to leave Seattle and we were all busy trying to go to the doctor and dentist one more time before our move? Well, one of mama's appointments was to go to the doctor and get a mammogram, which is basically pictures of my breasts to make sure that everything looks healthy. A few days after my mammogram appointment, I got a call from the doctor's office saying that they needed to get some better pictures. When I went back to get more pictures taken, the doctor found something that wasn't right. It is something called cancer and it's not good for cancer to stay in your body. The doctors don't know why I have cancer, but it is serious and it's important that I have a doctor take it out.

Once you guys started school, Papa and I went to some doctor appointments here in LA and the doctors made a plan to take the cancer out. That means that I will need to be in the hospital for a few days, but Nana will be coming to help take care of you while I'm away from home and Papa will go back and forth to check on me while I'm there.

After my surgery, the doctors will decide what is best to do next. There's a chance that I will need to take some medicine that will help keep the cancer from coming back, but the medicine could also make my hair fall out. This will be hard for me, but I want to do what is best to keep the cancer away. Like I said, we will know more after my surgery.

What questions do you have for me or Papa? If you don't have any right now, you can ask us questions any time.

That is the gist of what I shared with them. It was one of the hardest conversations of my life, but once I told them, there was a weight lifted off of me and now I could talk freely around them. It's amazing how all three kids could be hearing the same information, but have different reactions. Hope, who was nine at the time, was processing everything internally. You could see the wheels turning. Sophia was seven, and she was more outwardly concerned and asked a couple questions about logistics, and the ins and outs of surgery, and who was coming to stay with them. Zion was just five and he was very quiet as he heard the news. He came and sat next to me. I could tell that he knew this was serious, and he wanted to stay close in the face of uncertainty.

Nikita shared some from his perspective and added that they needed to be praying for me as this was a big deal. You could feel the weight of our words. After a few moments of quiet, Sophia said she had one more question, "Can we go to Target now?" I started cracking up. "Yes, let's go to Target." I think it was her way of saying something we were all feeling: *This is too heavy; can we move on to something fun and easy?* It was perfect timing and it was just what we all needed, a temporary break from the weight of our new reality.

Looking back, I'm not sure what was worse, waiting to tell them and suffering in silence, or dragging them into the foxhole with me and seeing the fear settle in. It's like playing, "Would you Rather" (one of my kids favorite games). Would you rather eat a sack of spider eggs, or take a shower with poisonous snakes? Tough call. At the end of the day, if I had to do it all over again, I would handle it the same way.

I know that your situation is not exactly like mine. Your kids might be different ages and they will have different needs than mine did.

Remember that God chose you to be their mama and you know what is best for them and your family. You know your kids better than anyone else.

As you head into your conversation with your kids, here are a few things to consider:

Days (or weeks if you have it) before, begin praying for your kids' hearts and that God would be preparing them to receive the news that you will share with them. Also pray for God to be the one speaking through you. He knows them even better than you do.

Even though I hate the word "cancer," it's important to use it instead of just saying, "Mama is sick." Younger kids like mine will have a hard time differentiating between being "sick" with a cold or cough, and "sick" with cancer. If they don't already know, let them know that cancer isn't contagious and they won't be able to get it from hugging you or being close to you.

If it feels overwhelming to use your own words to share with them, ask your husband or a trusted family member to tag team with you, or to tell them for you.

Even though this conversation will be hard for you and for them, they are a part of the family and they deserve to know (in a kids' version) what is going on. Kids are very intuitive and are probably already picking up on the new dynamic and stress that you are carrying around. Knowing the truth will help them understand what they are probably already sensing.

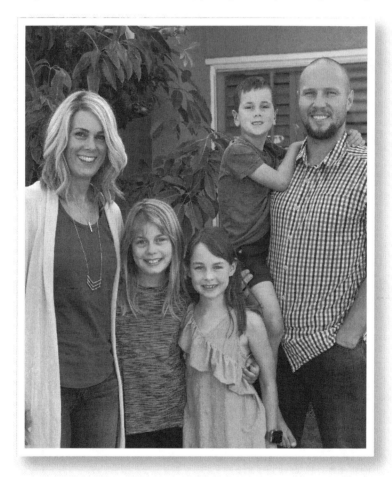

Remember that this is just a starting conversation. Everyone is different when finding out shocking news, so they may start firing questions right away, or they may be quietly processing in the moment, and their questions will come later. Be sure to let them know that they can ask you anything, anytime.

Depending on your child, he or she may need you (or your husband) to be the one to initiate with him or her and probe a bit. All of my kids ended up talking to me in different ways throughout that season, so have your antenna up and be ready to talk when they drop some clues that they might need time to process. To my surprise, Zion was the one who ended up talking to me the most and asking the most questions. When I would put him down at night he would ask questions about my wigs, my boobs, and if my hair would grow back blonde. He would share that he wished I hadn't lost my hair. Even though the things my kids asked or shared made me cry later, I am so thankful that they felt safe enough to invite me into their tender hearts.

Just like my kids, your kids are resilient. Even though this is not the way that you want them to grow into compassionate humans, God does not waste any circumstances or seasons. This time is no exception. He will use this valley you all are walking through to help them become more empathetic and in tune with the struggles that others are going through around them. Just like you, they will be able to put themselves in others' shoes and better understand the pain in someone else's eyes. They are tougher than you think and they are going to be okay; after all, they take after you.

Chapter 7
WHY SUFFERING?

Suffering. Sadly, there's no getting around it in this life. It would be nice to think that if you are a "good person" you can avoid the pain and suffering that this world dishes out. If I give the homeless enough food, if I'm a faithful friend and a caring neighbor, if I devote my life to serving God, maybe He will bless me and keep me from walking this well-worn path of suffering. I wish that's how it worked. I want to be able to control and manipulate God into giving me what I want, and avoiding the things that scare the crap out of me. I wish that I could be in control instead of God. Not that I necessarily think that I could do a better job, but if I were at the wheel, I would do my best to wrap myself and those I love with bubble wrap so that we wouldn't have to feel the pain that comes with being human.

Getting introduced to breast cancer hasn't helped with my doubts about God's goodness and love for me. In fact, it's reinforced the fact that something needs to be done about this God that allows people He "loves" to experience suffering and pain.

Growing up, my favorite Bible verse was Jeremiah 29:11 which says, "For I know the plans I have for you," declares the Lord. "Plans to prosper you and not to harm you, plans to give you hope and a future."[1] Sounds amazing, right? Who wouldn't choose this as their favorite Bible verse? Who doesn't want to prosper, have hope, a future, and not be harmed? This is what I was building my whole relationship with God upon. I do my part to follow Him and make Him known, and He does His job of prospering me, giving me hope, a future, and protecting me from harm. That sounds like a pretty good deal. You scratch my back, I'll scratch yours.

This symbiotic relationship with God was working very well for me until I got a call from my mom on August 23, 2008, telling me that my dad had suffered a stroke. To say that I was in complete shock would be a major understatement. Panic and fear washed over me and I felt paralyzed—and scared to death. The stroke was devastating, leaving my dad paralyzed on the right side and unable to communicate. The doctors who had been caring for him shared that if there were any improvements, they would likely come during the first year. So, I leaned into the Lord like I never had before, and decided to trust God had a plan and believe He would heal my dad.

In the end, God gave us five more years with my dad, but there were no improvements. I felt my heart begin to harden when I realized that it didn't matter how hard I prayed, if God didn't choose to heal him, my dad wouldn't be healed. I was devastated (again), as I came to terms with the fact that I would never hear my dad's voice again. I would never get to hang on his wisdom. I would never get to talk with him about the books we were reading or what God was teaching us. I was hurting and grieving as I realized that even though my dad was still here physically, I had lost the dad I had always known and I wanted him back.

Unfortunately, none of us can avoid the road of suffering. Similar to what I experienced when my dad got sick, when I was diagnosed, I initially leaned into God and turned to Him for help. I mean, who else could rescue me? I knew I needed help. My first prayer was that it wouldn't be cancer. But it was.

Then I prayed that I could "just" do a lumpectomy, but that wasn't an option. I prayed that it wouldn't be in my lymph nodes, but 2.2 millimeters said it was. When my tumor was sent out to test the genetic make-up, I prayed that it would determine that I wouldn't need chemo. As it turned out, the type of cancer I had responds well to chemo. Finally, I prayed that it wouldn't be the type of chemo that would cause me to lose my hair. It was.

When I first was diagnosed, I kept asking God, *Why me?* I was young for a breast cancer diagnosis and I had such major life changes ahead of me and so much upheaval in my world already. Why was God allowing this, and why was He allowing this at this time? It didn't seem to match up with my Jeremiah 29:11 life verse.

After giving God a piece of my mind for some time, my question morphed into a different one, *Why not me?* Who was I to think that out of all the pain and suffering that people were experiencing in the world, that I would somehow escape it? Or if I didn't think that this was a good time to go through this, when *would* be a good time? Is there ever a good time to find out you have breast cancer and that you need to go through extreme measures to save your life? No need to answer that one.

As I continued to wrestle with my suffering and with God, my question shifted yet again. I began to wonder, *Why would God even allow pain and suffering in this world?* Again, it just didn't match up with who I knew Him to be. Even as an imperfect mom, I would never let my child chase a ball into the street if I knew that a car was coming. I would do whatever I could to save and protect my child, so why wasn't God doing the same for His kids? Why would He even create us knowing that we would have to experience pain and suffering? I just couldn't fathom it. It felt pretty messed up.

Even though it's hard to not have all the answers (or any of them), I think it's important to ask the questions nonetheless. I'm like the kid in math class that wants to know why we have to learn this. I don't want to just learn a formula, but not know how I got that answer. I don't want to go through the motions with God either. I feel like if I know why it's important and what it's for, then I will be motivated to learn and be able to receive it more peacefully.

As I asked question after question and wove my way through the stages of grief, at some point I figuratively threw my hands in the air and had to accept the fact that on this side of heaven, I would never fully know why. I would never know why God had allowed my dad to experience a stroke. I would never know why I was diagnosed with cancer. This felt defeating, but I didn't have the emotional bandwidth to keep up with all the questions. I was emotionally spent.

One day not long after I tapped out, I felt like God revealed something to me so simple and obvious, but profound and helpful. I had the epiphany that there must be something I didn't know yet. Assuming that God really is who the Bible says He is....loving, kind, merciful, just, and yet He would allow this pain and suffering to enter my world and yours, then there must be something that I couldn't see. There must be something He knows that I can't yet comprehend. You see, we have only seen and experienced the first part of the story, but He knows the rest. He can see the bigger picture and how everything has purpose and meaning, even our suffering.

Like the well-known tapestry metaphor that we've all heard, one side is messy and chaotic, but the other is perfectly beautiful. I realized that I had been fixating on the mess and confusion on the back side, and I was paralyzed and overwhelmed by the chaos of criss-crossed strings, knots, and dead-ends. It felt like too much. As I found myself stuck and tangled in the brokenness of my life, I couldn't help but view God as broken and messed up, too. I was looking at my circumstances and determining who God was through that lens.

Instead of allowing our circumstances to define who God is, what if we choose to see God through the truths that the Bible says about who He is? Those are the things that never change. If we are viewing Him through our circumstances and suffering, of course He will look like a calloused and uncaring God. And each time our circumstances change, our view of God changes. Like it says in Hebrews 12:2, we must consider, "... keeping our eyes on Jesus, the champion who initiates and perfects our faith. Because of the joy awaiting him, he endured the cross, disregarding its shame."[2] Instead of focusing on the circumstances around us that are here today and gone tomorrow, what if we keep our eyes on Him, the one who will never change?

Through our suffering we become more like Christ and share in the suffering He experienced. He understands our pain and confusion, because He also endured suffering. He is not a God who is distant and protected. He came near to face the disappointment, obstacles, and pain we experience. He also draws near to us through His Spirit to guide, comfort, and bring, "peace that passes all understanding."³ This makes me want to trust Him. He doesn't just allow our suffering, He stepped into it and joined us when He was nailed to a cross and carried the weight of suffering for us. He didn't have to do that, but He chose to.

I still hate the fact that I don't fully understand, and that He doesn't answer all of my why's here on earth. But the fact that He promises to walk with me through the uncertainties and anguish of my pain and suffering, that shows me His heart. He is not the friend who means well but says something really insensitive because He's not acquainted with suffering. Instead, He is the one who has walked the path of suffering, and He understands the heartache that comes with it. He knows when to listen, when to cry with you, when to make you laugh, or take your mind off of it all. He understands your heartache, because He felt the weight of it as He hung on the cross. He felt the weight of the brokenness of our world and our bodies. So as you weep and mourn the loss of your old life and begin to accept the fact that cancer is now part of your story, trust that Jesus is drawing near. He is with you. You are not alone.

LOVED

CaringBridge Journal entry by Tanya Motorin
September 24, 2018

A few years ago, Nikita and the kids gave me a special gift for Mother's Day. I wear it most every day. It's a necklace and vertical pendant with the word "Loved" inscribed on it. It is precious to me not only because it's from my sweet family, but because it's a daily reminder to me that I am loved. Loved by my husband. Loved by my kids. Loved by God.

Even though I already knew that I was loved before I ever put on the necklace, each day when I reach behind my head and secure the necklace around my neck, I am reminded again of this beautiful love that covers me. Even when I don't feel lovely, or my circumstances seem dark, I know that I am loved.

This picture of putting on love reminds me of what the Israelites were commanded to do when they were given the second set of stone tablets in Deuteronomy 11[4]. They weren't commanded to just, "Love the Lord and obey His commandments," but as verse 18 says to, "Fix these words of mine in your hearts and minds; tie them as symbols on your hands and bind them on your foreheads." Why did God want them to do all this? When I read this in the past, I always just thought that the Israelites were clueless and couldn't remember God's commandments. However, when I was rereading this passage this morning, verse 8 stood out to me which says, "Observe therefore all the commands I am giving you today, <u>so that you may have the strength</u> to go in and take over the land that you are crossing the Jordan to possess."

That feels different to me. That tells me that God's words breathe life and give strength for the journey ahead. His words were equipping them and empowering them for what only God knew they would face. It was true for the Israelites, and it's true for me. I can choose to believe that God's words are just words without any power, or I can trust that they are breathing life into me, sustaining me, and giving me all that I need as I come face-to-face with cancer.

I've had friends and family tell me that they hate that I have to go through this. I hate it, too. I wish I could go back to July 24th and rewrite this chapter of my story, but I can't. I hate this, but I am choosing to believe that even though my circumstances are awful and God doesn't feel very safe right now, I know that He is good and His promises are true because they are the only thing sustaining me. He is always true to who He says He is.

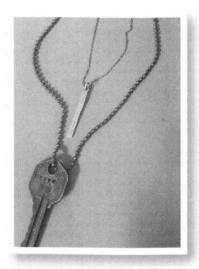

I got another necklace last week from a 4-year-old. I was having brunch at a friend's house and her son was wearing a chain with a key hanging from it. I told him that I liked it and asked him what it said. He held the key up and I read the word "Brave" on it. Then, with the gentle encouragement from his mom, he took off the chain and gave it to me. My eyes welled up with tears, because I so desperately want to be brave right now, but I just can't, I'm too scared. It's too much to bear. Then, as I looked down to see my new "Brave" necklace hanging below my "Loved" necklace, it dawned on me that I don't have to be brave. It's not about me. His love makes me brave.

Chapter 8

A DIFFERENT KIND OF LOVE

At some point during the year when I was undergoing surgery, chemo, and radiation, I reread the story of Lazarus. Even though I had read this story many times before, it was as if I was reading it for the first time. I always need to be reminded of God's love, but I especially did during that year from hell. Like Mary, Martha, and Lazarus, I needed to know that when everything around me was starting to crumble, His love was still there. Steadfast. Faithful. Powerful. Reading the story of Lazarus reminded me of this steady love I had known, and it gave me eyes to see God's love in new ways. Let's take a look at it together.

John 11 NIV
The Death of Lazarus

1 Now a man named Lazarus was sick. He was from Bethany, the village of Mary and her sister Martha. 2 (This Mary, whose brother Lazarus now lay sick, was the same one who poured perfume on the Lord and wiped his feet with her hair.) 3 So the sisters sent word to Jesus, "Lord, the one you love is sick." 4 When he heard this, Jesus said, "This sickness will not end in death. No, it is for God's glory so that God's Son may be glorified through it." 5 Now Jesus loved Martha and her sister and Lazarus. 6 So when he heard that Lazarus was sick, he stayed where he was two more days, 7 and then he said to his disciples, "Let us go back to Judea." 8 "But Rabbi," they said, "a short while ago the Jews there tried to stone you, and yet you are going back?" 9 Jesus answered, "Are there not twelve hours of daylight? Anyone who walks in the daytime will not stumble, for they see by this world's light. 10 It is when a person walks at night that they stumble, for they have no light." 11 After he had said this, he went on to tell them, "Our friend Lazarus has fallen asleep; but I am going there to wake him up." 12 His disciples replied, "Lord, if he sleeps, he will get better." 13 Jesus had been speaking of his death, but his disciples thought he meant natural sleep. 14 So then he told them plainly, "Lazarus is dead, 15 and for your sake I am glad I was not there, so that you may believe. But let us go to him." 16 Then Thomas (also known as Didymus[a]) said to the rest of the disciples, "Let us also go, that we may die with him."

Jesus Comforts the Sisters of Lazarus

17 On his arrival, Jesus found that Lazarus had already been in the tomb for four days.

18 Now Bethany was less than two miles[b] from Jerusalem, 19 and many Jews had come to Martha and Mary to comfort them in the loss of their brother. 20 When Martha heard that Jesus was coming, she went out to meet him, but Mary stayed at home.

21 "Lord," Martha said to Jesus, "if you had been here, my brother would not have died. 22 But I know that even now God will give you whatever you ask." 23 Jesus said to her, "Your brother will rise again." 24 Martha answered, "I know he will rise again in the resurrection at the last day." 25 Jesus said to her, "I am the resurrection and the life. The one who believes in me will live, even though they die; 26 and whoever lives by believing in me will never die. Do you believe this?" 27 "Yes, Lord," she replied, "I believe that you are the Messiah, the Son of God, who is to come into the world."

28 After she had said this, she went back and called her sister Mary aside. "The Teacher is here," she said, "and is asking for you." 29 When Mary heard this, she got up quickly and went to him. 30 Now Jesus had not yet entered the village, but was still at the place where Martha had met him. 31 When the Jews who had been with Mary in the house, comforting her, noticed how quickly she got up and went out, they followed her, supposing she was going to the tomb to mourn there. 32 When Mary reached the place where Jesus was and saw him, she fell at his feet and said, "Lord, if you had been here, my brother would not have died." 33 When Jesus saw her weeping, and the Jews who had come along with her also weeping, he was deeply moved in spirit and troubled. 34 "Where have you laid him?" he asked. "Come and see, Lord," they replied. 35 Jesus wept. 36 Then the Jews said, "See how he loved him!" 37 But some of them said, "Could not he who opened the eyes of the blind man have kept this man from dying?"

Jesus Raises Lazarus From the Dead

38 Jesus, once more deeply moved, came to the tomb. It was a cave with a stone laid across the entrance. 39 "Take away the stone," he said. "But, Lord," said Martha, the sister of the dead man, "by this time there is a bad odor, for he has been there four days." 40 Then Jesus said, "Did I not tell you that if you believe, you will see the glory of God?" 41 So they took away the stone. Then Jesus looked up and said, "Father, I thank you that you have heard me. 42 I knew that you always hear me, but I said this for the benefit of the people standing here, that they may believe that you sent me."

43 When he had said this, Jesus called in a loud voice, "Lazarus, come out!" 44 The dead man came out, his hands and feet wrapped with strips of linen, and a cloth around his face. Jesus said to them, "Take off the grave clothes and let him go."[1]

Let's start by looking at verses 3 and 5. In these verses it becomes pretty obvious that the writer wants us to know that Lazarus and his sisters were loved by Jesus. Not only that, he wants us to know that they knew it. He writes, "So the sisters sent word to Jesus, 'Lord, the one you love is sick.'" This is significant because the writer, John, wants us to see the firm foundation that Jesus had laid in their lives ahead of time so that they would be able to withstand the devastation that would come later. They needed to be rooted in Christ's love in order to remain standing when the floor dropped out from underneath them.

If you take a look at verse 6, we see that God's love doesn't always make sense. John just got done telling us in verse 5 how much Jesus loved Lazarus and his sisters, so in my mind it would make sense if verse 6 said, "So when he heard that Lazarus, his friend that he loved was sick, Jesus dropped everything and came as quickly as he could to be with Lazarus and heal him." That makes more sense, right? It makes sense to me because that's what I would do if one of my people were sick, hurting, or dying. Like when my daughter, Sophia, was six and she fell out of a tree that her and my son were climbing. I didn't slowly walk over, mildly curious to see if she was breathing. I sprinted around the huge evergreen tree so fast that my flip flops flew off because I had to make sure my baby was okay. My mama bear instincts kicked in and there was no one who could have kept me from her. But as the account of Lazarus unfolds, we don't see Jesus pick up his robe and run so fast that his sandals fall off. Instead, John starts verse 6 with a three letter word, *yet*. "Yet, when he heard that Lazarus was sick, he stayed where he was two more days."

Yet? Are you kidding me? I would have felt so betrayed if Jesus had purposefully waited two more days. Mary and Martha were reaching out to Him because they needed Him and they knew that He was the only one who could help. It says right there in the text that Jesus loved Mary, Martha, and Lazarus, but it would have been difficult for me to understand how waiting two more days could communicate love. As I read this part, I thought, *"No, Jesus, this is not the time to dawdle. The friend that you love needs you. Whatever you are doing, set it aside and get yourself to Bethany. There's not much time to spare."*

I think I can relate so much to the story of Lazarus because when I got my breast cancer diagnosis, I was confused, too. That's not really a strong enough word actually. I was in disbelief. Dumbfounded. Pissed off. It didn't make sense. I wondered, *"How could this be happening?"* I had grown up in the church and had walked closely with God since I was ten years old when I asked Him to be in my life. So, I knew God loved me, but His love had never looked like this before. It didn't feel like love and I didn't like it. I still don't. His actions didn't make sense. Why wasn't He doing what I asked Him to do? Why didn't He choose to heal me instead of allowing cancer to enter my body and chaos to enter my life? How could allowing me to get cancer be demonstrating His love for me? How could He allow three of my friends to recently die of cancer?

It's been a few years since my diagnosis and unfortunately, I still don't have the answers to any of these questions. If you're in the midst of the valley of the shadow of death, I know that you must have a long detailed list of questions, too. I hate this for me and I hate it for you. I wish that God's love was more predictable. More of a formula to follow like a+b=c. Let's give it a try...I follow You all of my life (not perfectly, but the best I can) + I pray and bring the hard stuff to You = You make it all better by removing any pain, suffering, discomfort, or sickness.

Like me, both Mary and Martha pushed back in verses 21 and 32. They both questioned Jesus, saying, "Lord, if you had been here, my brother would not have died." They didn't understand how he could love them, and love Lazarus, and yet choose to stay where He was two more days, especially when He knew that His friend was dying. When it really mattered, He didn't come in time.

I wish I could say that I've cracked the code. However, I still have questions, fears, and doubts rumbling around in my head and heart. What I have settled on is the fact that, even though I can't avoid pain and suffering in this world, I'm not alone in it. Not only does Jesus see my suffering, He joins me in it. In verses 33, 35, and 38, we see a glimpse of Jesus' heart for those He loves. Verse 33 says, "He was deeply moved in spirit and troubled." Verse 35 says, "He wept." And then in verse 38 it says, "Jesus, once more deeply moved..."

Not only is Jesus with us as we walk this road of suffering, He takes time to enter into our pain, connect with our hearts, and grieve with us before making things right. Before He mends, He draws near. Before He makes us whole again and redeems the brokenness, He first sits with us in the heartbreak. Instead of rushing to the rescue, He grieves with Mary and Martha when they thought that He was too late. He wept when their hearts were broken over the loss of their brother, because His heart was broken, too.

He does the same for us. He draws near and grieves with us because we are not yet able to understand or see how He could possibly redeem and restore all that has been lost. Don't you think that instead of spending thirty-three years walking this earth, Jesus could have come down and immediately died on the cross? He could have immediately gotten down to business, but instead He waited. He chose to become a baby, go through the awkward stages of growing up, experience the highs and lows of life in this broken world, to walk in our shoes. Then after thirty-three years, He decided to take our pain and suffering, and begin the process of redemption. He is a God that draws near. He doesn't give us advice or encouragement from the sideline. Instead, He put on flesh and became like us. He was broken—like us.

Jesus did the same for Mary and Martha. After meeting them in their pain and anguish and then extending empathy, Jesus did what only He can do. He brought Lazarus back to life. Not just for them, but to display His power.

After eight months of diagnosis, surgery and treatment, I felt about as dead as Lazarus in the tomb. I was exhausted not only physically, but also emotionally and spiritually. I had the life sucked out of me, and the only thing left was bottom of the barrel grit. It helped on some days, but most days, it just wasn't enough. Not to be dramatic, but I felt like I was in the tomb. I was buried in the depths and it seemed as though there wasn't even a hint of daylight. It was the darkest night of my soul. I couldn't see what He might possibly be doing. It was too dark to even squint and try to make out a figure in the darkness.

As I read in my NIV Study Bible notes from the account of Lazarus, I learned that at the time, people believed that after someone had died, their soul would hang out around them for three more days. So, even after they died, there was this hope that they could come back to life, as long as their soul was still there. Hence the reason why the sisters were so desperate to have Jesus come immediately. But this detail was not lost on Jesus. He wasn't just preoccupied and unable to get to them quickly. I am confident that He purposefully waited to come because He loved them. But how? He knew that if He came right away, Lazarus might still be alive when He arrived and He could heal him and God would get the glory. Or, if He waited a day and arrived after Lazarus had died, He could raise Him from the dead and God could get even more glory. But by waiting two days plus the time it took to travel there, it had actually been four days since Lazarus had died, so there was no hope that his soul would be able to enter back into his body. He wasn't just dead. He was really dead. (Is that a thing?) So, when Jesus showed up four days "late," not only would God get the most glory when He healed Lazarus, but Mary and Martha and the others present, would also have their faith stretched beyond what they understood. Not only would He heal their brother, but He would do it in a way that no one knew was possible.

Even though I don't like it, Lazarus' story has taught me that it's not all about me. Yes, Jesus loves me and cares for me so deeply, but because His love is the kind of love described in 1 Corinthians 13[2], He doesn't want me to stay in the place where I've been. Yes, it may feel comfy and cozy, but that is not my purpose here on earth. My purpose is to reflect Him and to give God the MOST glory. I've begged God to allow me to grow closer to Him through podcasts and great sermons on Sunday (and I do), but the reality is, I grow the most and begin to look most like Him when I go through the fire of life's challenges.

Why? Because fire makes me moldable and malleable to be used by Him and for Him. Fire pulls out the impurities. If Jesus learned obedience through suffering, why wouldn't I too? I'm not just here to get a great house, marry a hot guy, raise wonderful kids, and get the most likes on Instagram. We were made by God, for God, and, as Psalm 23[3] reminds us, sometimes He will make us lie down in green pastures, but other times, He will walk with us through the valley of the shadow of death.

PART 2
Your Story

I can't emphasize enough how important it has been for me to have space to take a step back and acknowledge the hell that I've been through. Writing down my story has been a powerful piece in my healing process as it's allowed me to continue grieving all that I've lost as well as giving me room to peel back the layers of what I am still holding. If you're like me, I didn't have the bandwidth in the midst of surgery and treatment to begin writing my story, but whenever I had an idea in the middle of the night, I would add it to the notes section on my phone in hopes that I would have the strength to circle back and tease it out later.

Now that you've heard my story, I want to encourage you to write yours down, too. Whether you decide to write your own book or just jot your thoughts and feelings down from time to time, it is important to begin unpacking the depths of what you've been through and all that you are currently experiencing. Sometimes there aren't words to describe the deep valleys and heartache you've experienced. I know. It's horrible, and no one should ever have to endure what you're going through, and yet, here you are. If nothing less, when you are ready, I hope this can be a healing exercise to help you pull out some of the emotional toxins that come with this journey. If it's helpful, get out your computer or buy a journal to jot your thoughts down. Either way, your story is worth telling.

Essentials For The Journey

Before we get any further, I want to share a few "must haves" that you'll need to "pack" for this journey. I'm one of those people that has different packing lists saved on my computer for different types of trips. If I'm going camping with my family, the things I'll need are very different than if I'm going on an anniversary getaway with my hubby. When I'm going someplace I've never been before, I try to pick the brain of someone who's been there. I want to figure out what I need and what I should leave at home. The last thing one needs is too much baggage.

So, this section is to help you be as prepared as possible for the journey ahead. I wish so badly that you were going on a fun vacation and I was sharing with you what you'll need for your adventure. This is a journey you never signed up for and you have no desire to be on. If I could wave a magic wand and make it all go away, I would. The best I can do is be here for you by sharing some helpful hints and my thoughts on what to "pack" since I've already been down this path. Just because I've travelled down this road doesn't make me an expert, but I would like to share five essentials that were so helpful for me.

Here's what I think you'll need:

1. FIND YOUR A-TEAM
2. MAKE SPACE FOR GRIEF
3. GIVE YOURSELF PERMISSION
4. BE KIND TO YOURSELF
5. CELEBRATE ALONG THE WAY

Chapter 9

FIND YOUR A-TEAM

So much of who I am today has been influenced by the lessons I've learned on the soccer field. My first team was named, "The Force" and with my fellow five-year-olds, we followed the ball around like a cluster of piranhas hungry for a goal. Over the years I grew as a player and learned volumes about what it meant to be a part of a team, especially the importance of listening to my teammates as well as working together to get the win. Not only did I learn from my teammates, I also had to take the input of my coaches and trainers, and make adjustments accordingly. My teammates and I learned how to depend on each other to accomplish our goal as a unit. Together we carried the pressure when we were behind, and we celebrated together after a hard-fought victory. I couldn't win on my own; I needed them and they needed me.

Similarly, you've entered into a fierce battle and even though you are the one who had or has cancer in your body, this battle is not just yours. You cannot do this alone, even if you wanted to. There are others around you who will battle with you. Some "teammates" will be there by default (husband, kids, extended family), and others you will need to handpick, because they will each bring a certain skill set or expertise that you need. This is the team of people who will have your back and help carry you through this horrible time.

This team that you form will be much like the men who brought their paralyzed friend to Jesus because they heard that He was healing people (Mark 2:1-12)[1]. Who knows how long they had to carry him to get to the house where Jesus was, but when they got there, they weren't able to reach Jesus because of the crowds who had also come to be healed. Instead of hanging their heads and heading home, they cut a hole in the roof and lowered the man to Jesus. In Mark 2:5 it says, "When Jesus saw their faith, he said to the paralyzed man, 'Son, your sins are forgiven.'" Jesus highlighted the faith of the man's friends and, as a result, Jesus healed the man and he ended up picking up his mat and walking home that night.

These are the kind of people you need on your team. People who won't give up on you. Friends who will keep carrying you until you get the healing and care you need. No matter how badly the man wanted to be healed, he didn't have what was required to get himself healed. He needed his four friends to pick up a corner of his mat and carry him to the One who could heal him.

For some of you, it is reassuring to know that there are others speaking encouragement, offering their service, helping to carry the load, and patching you up. But for others, it might be completely out of your comfort zone to ask for help or allow yourself to depend on people, especially during such a vulnerable time. I get that. I mean, after all, we've learned to be strong, independent women who pull ourselves up by our bootstraps, right? Right. But battling cancer is not an individual sport. You will crumble quickly if you try to go it alone. You need people who love and care for you to surround you during this time—and after. You need your teammates. It's actually a "win-win" because you need the help and people who love you deeply are wanting to ease your pain. They wish there was something they could do to help. Let them.

Okay, so now that we've established that you can't do this alone, it's time to choose your team. Let me remind you that you are in fact going into battle, so do not settle for anyone but the best beside you. If you're having second thoughts, move on to a better fit. Think back to dodgeball at lunch recess. You are the captain, so you get to pick the best, because you're here to win. Cancer is going down.

DOCTORS

Obviously you need top-notch doctors to care for you during this time. Do your research online and ask others who have been through this journey who they've used and why. Make sure they are brilliant and outstanding at what they do, but you also need doctors that make you feel at ease. You want doctors that see you. Not just as a patient, but also as a person. I feel so cared for when my doctors remember details about my life beyond cancer...what I do, how many kids I have, where I'm from, etc. Sometimes it's the little things that make a BIG difference.

The doctors you'll need are:

1. Breast surgeon
2. Plastic surgeon
3. Oncologist
4. Radiation Oncologist (possibly)
5. Primary Care Physician

I chose to have all of my doctors within the UCLA system not only because they were outstanding, but I also wanted it to be easy for them to communicate with one another and not have to wait for images or results to come in from a different medical system.

Even though all the doctors are equally important for your care, I would say that choosing your oncologist and your primary care physician will be the most important. The oncologist is vital because he or she is the one that you will be spending the most time with for chemo, blood work, follow ups, etc. You want to make sure you feel that you are in good hands. The primary care physician is invaluable because he or she is the one who will need to be the conductor of this whole care "orchestra." I would suggest seeing her every 2-3 months for the first year or so. This will keep you on her radar and she will be better in tune with how you are doing physically and emotionally. It makes a world of difference to have someone who sees the bigger picture with you and oversees all of your care so that you aren't just talking to a bunch of specialists who only specialize in their particular field.

Before you get too far into this journey, go to an office supply store and get a big binder with some folders, dividers, and a pouch. Make a tab for each doctor you have and keep any notes you take there, as well as "after appointment" summaries. I also put business cards and other useful information in the pouch. For me, this was a quick and easy way to organize and access all of my medical notes and paperwork for future reference.

CARINGBRIDGE COMMUNICATOR

It was a really big step for me when I decided to create a CaringBridge site[2] because when my dad had his stroke, we used CaringBridge as our main form of communication to his friends and our extended family. Even though it was such a blessing to be able to update everyone all at once, each time I would log on to write an update, I couldn't believe that this had really happened to my dad.

It was difficult for me to make my own CaringBridge site because, not only was I flooded with emotions and memories of my dad's long-term illness, I was now faced with the reality that I had something serious enough going on in my body that warranted my own CaringBridge site. At the same time, I was so overwhelmed trying to text everyone individually, it quickly became apparent to me that I needed a place to update people regarding my medical developments, how to pray, and how to help.

Once I mustered up the courage to create my CaringBridge site and began sending the link to people so they could follow my journey, a huge burden was lifted off my shoulders. It meant so much that people cared enough to want to stay informed about my journey, but it meant even more that I could keep them updated in a way that wasn't burdensome for me. If you don't want to write your own updates, creating a CaringBridge site could be a good job for a family member or trusted friend.

While I was in the hospital, my sister posted a couple updates to keep everyone in the loop the day of my surgery as well as during my recovery. Having her update people during that time gave Nikita one less responsibility to carry while he was going back and forth between home and the hospital that week. Later, Nikita posted updates as well. Once I felt up to it,

I continued using CaringBridge for at least a year after my diagnosis. Not only was it a great way to keep people informed, but it became another avenue for me to write and process many of the emotions and struggles I faced during that time. Having this cathartic outlet was a key component of my emotional and spiritual healing.

MEAL TRAIN

Meal Train[3], is a great way for people to sign up online to bring meals for you and your family. My sister offered to set up a site for us which provided delicious meals for our family while also giving people a practical way to help. This was a helpful option for out-of-town friends to send some love via UberEats or send a gift card for one of our favorite restaurants. I was especially grateful for this service since cooking meals for our family was a job that generally fell on me. Meal Train helped take some of weight off of my shoulders.

> *Practical tip:* Have people sign up for meals every other day so your fridge doesn't get overcrowded with leftovers and new meals.

PRAYER WARRIORS

Even though this is a physical and emotional battle, it is a spiritual battle as well. There were so many times during this season that I questioned my faith and the faithfulness of God. Because of this, I not only needed people caring for my medical and physical needs, I needed people helping to cover my spiritual needs as well. During this time I would try to post on CaringBridge every week or two to let people know what was going on and how they could be praying. I can't tell you what a privilege it was to have hundreds of people interceding for me on a regular basis.

In addition to posting my prayer requests, I also had an inner circle of friends and family who were praying for the daily things I was struggling with and the raw emotions I couldn't always share on CaringBridge.

Some of these people I chose because I know their hearts for God and for me, but others chose me. They would faithfully text, call, or send me a video message on Marco Polo[4] (even if I didn't respond right away or ever), or they sent cards sharing encouraging verses and prayers.

There were times when I didn't have the strength to believe, so these friends believed for me and reminded me that I was not alone in this battle. Whether they are new friends or old, it is vital to have a team of people interceding on your behalf.

EMPATHETIC FRIENDS

There were also friends I turned to when I needed someone to cry with and give me a huge dose of empathy. I didn't need them to try to fix me or the problem, I just needed them to climb into the pit with me and try to put themselves in my shoes and to imagine what I must be feeling. It was absolutely life-giving to have a safe space to let it all out, have a good cry together, and then move on to face the day.

TRAIL GUIDES

Our family enjoys hiking in the Santa Monica Mountains not far from where we live, but I wouldn't call myself an avid hiker. However, I do know how important it can be, especially when going on a bigger, more serious hike, to have a trail guide. Someone who knows the way, the things you should bring, and what to do in difficult or unknown territory. The same is true when it comes to this journey with cancer. It's absolutely vital to have a breast cancer "trail guide" to help you along the way. The only prerequisite for this guide is that she has either already travelled this road, or she is a little bit ahead of you. What a blessing these guides are. They know better than anyone what you will likely be facing because they have already been there. These guides are familiar with the "terrain" like no one else.

If you haven't found a guide yet, my hope is that this book will serve as a guide for you, but nothing will replace the human interaction you can have with someone who has walked in your shoes. God raised up several guides for me, some of them I had known for years, and others I met once I started my journey. All of them offered a listening ear, helpful advice and shared with me the must-haves that I would need for my journey. Thank you Melinda, Tracy, Lisa, Debra, Shannon, Christine, Susan, Pam, Ligaya, Kim, Laurie, and E.

FUN FRIENDS

Fun friends are a must for this journey. People who know what's going on, but don't need to ask a million questions because they know I'll bring it up if I want to talk about it. They are there to bring smiles, companionship and lots of laughter.

While I was going through treatment one of the moms from my son's Kindergarten class texted a few of us about a mom's night out. I responded (immediately), "This is exactly what I need right now!" I almost felt normal that night as I got dressed up, enjoyed delicious food, great wine, and some deep laughter. Best part of the evening? No one mentioned one thing about cancer. It was the best gift I had received in a long time.

PAY IT FORWARD

Now that you are walking on this path, this qualifies you to be a trail guide for someone else. Depending on where you are on the journey, you may not feel as though you have anything to give to anyone else, but once you start to feel stronger, you'll know when it's time to open yourself up to others who may need you.

Since going through breast cancer, God crossed my path with many women who are in various stages of their breast cancer journey. I've been able to care for them by praying, sharing about my journey, and being present when nothing makes sense.

You may not feel as though you are equipped to help other women in any way, but you'd be surprised. Sometimes it's just comforting to know that you're not alone. Even giving other women a visual of what they could look or feel like in six months, a year, or ten years, is reassuring to know that it won't always be this hard or quite as scary.

All of these teammates are different, yet each one offers a unique perspective and much needed assistance. There may be others that you'll need that I didn't list, but the important thing is to find the team that's right for you. Remember you are the captain, and your team will help you kick cancer's butt, so don't settle for anything less than the best.

Chapter 10

MAKING SPACE FOR GRIEF

Grief. I know some think there's no point in grieving, after all, it can't bring back all that was lost, postponed, or changed. However, if I've learned anything from my time in counseling over the years, I've come to recognize the importance of grieving and acknowledging all that has been lost. When I was in the thick of it after my diagnosis, all I wanted was to put it all behind me. I wanted to get healthy, keep moving forward, and never take a second glance in my rearview mirror.

However, the irony of it all is that I had to sit in the mess and acknowledge my traveling companions—grief and sorrow—before I could begin to move forward. Sure, it initially seems easier to ignore the sadness and disappointment, turn on Netflix, and eat some Cheetos. But that Band-Aid only works for so long and the elephant in the room doesn't go away just because you're ignoring it. Sooner or later we need to make eye contact with the wreckage, acknowledge how much we miss life before cancer, and grieve. We must get in the boxing arena and go some rounds with grief. In doing so, we are giving God an invitation to begin healing the wounds inflicted by our shattering.

So, what do you do with all that has been stirred up inside by this life- altering diagnosis? Unfortunately it's too big to ignore, escape, or sweep under the rug. Since the broken pieces won't mend themselves, we need to begin to grieve what has been lost. No one likes to enter into grief, I get it. It's associated with death, suffering, and pain. It's a horrible place to visit, much less somewhere you want to camp out. Grief is no joke. It's exhausting, physically, emotionally, and spiritually. And yet it is necessary. We need to grieve in order to fully heal. And no matter where you are in your cancer journey, you (like me) also need to continue to grieve the loss of the life you knew before cancer became a part of your story. We need to pay tribute to that which was lost when cancer came and disrupted our imperfect, but beautiful lives.

If you're someone who likes to always look on the bright side of things and perhaps you have the tendency of shoving the unpleasant things into the bulging closet in the hallway, you may have no clue where to even begin. Maybe you are feeling that your brokenness is just too deep, and it will be too painful to "go there." It can be tempting to pull yourself up by your bootstraps (because that's what strong women do, right?). But unfortunately, when we turn our backs on the hard things we might buy ourselves a bit of time, but ultimately, they will come back in another way, shape, or form to wreak more havoc.

So, if you can't avoid it, how can you begin to sort through the emotional wreckage? If you are not familiar with the five stages of grief, this is a good place to start. I'm not an expert on grief, but I have experienced grief as a process, not an event. It's cyclical, not linear. I wish that it was something like a shot at the doctor's office, or a bee sting that is uncomfortable for a moment, but then it's behind us.

Instead, Elisabeth Kubler-Ross describes grief in stages: denial, anger, bargaining, depression, and acceptance.[5] It's important to note that these stages aren't just boxes to check off so you can move to the next stage. As you grieve, you may experience some acceptance one day, and then feel anger and depression the next. I wish that grief was more predictable, but from my experience it can be messy, drawn-out, and with more layers than I'd prefer.

As you grieve, I've found it's important to not compare your journey to other women who are grieving and processing in a different way. This was my pitfall at times. I would look at others I talked to on this journey and see their experience as "normal," and then wonder why I wasn't able to respond in the same way or be where they were emotionally. Shame was the last thing I needed on top of my pain and grief. I want to encourage you that regardless of which stage of grief you find yourself in, it's okay. Grieving is a process that is unique and different for each of us walking on this path. Sometimes it can be a painfully slow and uncomfortable process, but because there's not a set timeline to follow, or a formula you can plug numbers into, you have permission to be right where you are. Your grief journey is unique to you so there's no judgment when you find yourself in one stage longer than you expected, or when you revisit a stage you thought you were done with. You've never gone through this before, so you have permission to be a potluck of emotions.

In this chapter, I wanted to help normalize what you are going through, but also give you some tracks to run on, especially if you're feeling hesitant about leaning into your grief. Here are some baby steps that might be helpful in getting you started. Okay, I just chuckled to myself out loud because I thought of the movie, *What About Bob?*[26] If you have no idea what I'm talking about, maybe that should be your first baby step. After watching the movie and having a good laugh, now it's time to get down to business. Here are some baby steps that may be helpful in your grieving process:

>>>**On a 3x5 card or Post-it Note, write down why you are stepping into the grieving process.** If you need to start with, "Because Tanya told me to," that's fine. Then, take some time to think about why you want or need to move through this pain and heartbreak.

Maybe you can write down your kids' names or your husband's, reminding you that your mental health not only affects you, but those around you. After you write something on your card, I want you to put it on your bathroom mirror or in a place that you will see often. Let this serve as a reminder that though this path of grief is painful, remembering your "why" is a vital piece that will help propel you towards a healthier place.

>>>**Make a list of all the things that have been lost, ruined, or changed because because of your diagnosis.** This might feel depressing, but it's necessary to acknowledge what has changed because of breast cancer. We often want to minimize what we are going through to convince ourselves that it's not a big deal. I hate to break it to you, but cancer is a big freaking deal. Keep getting more paper to add to your list if needed. Include little stuff and big stuff. It all matters.

>>>**Write a letter to your old self (pre-diagnosis).** Write whatever you want. If you need ideas, maybe include telling yourself what you miss, what you wish, what you are sad about. Or do you need to let yourself know that this isn't because of something you did, it's just something that happened?

>>>**Keep a journal**. Not a diary that talks about what you did today, but a space to express how you are feeling and why. Sometimes you know that you feel crappy, but you don't know why. Give yourself space to unpack what's going on beneath the surface. Some days you'll feel pretty good and you should celebrate that! Other days will be rough and you'll need a place to process everything you are holding. If you believe in God, this would be a great place to tell Him what's on your heart. The things you are praising Him for and the things that still feel scary. Don't hold back. He can handle it.

>>>**Join a breast cancer support group, find a counselor, or connect in some way with other women who have also walked this path.** In 2021, *The Journal of the National Comprehensive Cancer Network* conducted a study on the effect of a Christian-based support group on the emotional health of cancer survivors and caregivers. They found that 91% of the cancer patients, survivors, and caregivers who participated in a Christian-based support program felt their anxiety had improved or greatly improved while they were in the program, and depression levels decreased by 79%.[7]

Since I didn't feel comfortable pouring out my heart to a room full of women that I didn't know, I sought out one-on-one counseling. I am thankful that my counselor is also a breast cancer survivor so I know she gets it. I also enjoy going on walks with my neighbor who is another breast cancer survivor. Talking on the phone or meeting with other friends who have walked this path before me has been helpful as well. It's good to be able to talk to women who "get it." Even though you won't find someone with a diagnosis or treatment exactly like yours, other breast cancer survivors understand what it feels like to have their world shaken to the core. Be real and honest with them. You don't have to have it altogether, they understand the ups and down because they've been there.

>>>**Allow yourself as much time as you need to grieve and heal.** There's no timeline for grief. Just because someone else's journey has looked different than yours, it doesn't mean that they did it right and you're doing it wrong. Give yourself freedom to be where you're at. I know it's uncomfortable and you just want to get through it, but grieving is cathartic and necessary to sit in until you sense it's time to move forward.

>>>**Find a good book or podcast that helps you unpack what you're going through.** I'll be honest, I didn't find one that really hit the spot for me (maybe that's why I decided to write my own book). However, the book of Job in the Bible was helpful for me at one point, and also Joseph's story in Genesis. Some other books that were helpful in some ways were, *Don't Waste Your Cancer by* John Piper, *It's Not Fair* by Melanie Dale, *Pretty Sick* by Caitlin M. Kiernan, and *Walking with God Through Pain and Suffering* by Tim Keller.[8]

>>>**Practice gratitude.** It doesn't take long to jot a quick note about something that you are thankful for. A friend of mine gave me a beautiful journal when I was going through treatment and I decided to turn it into my thankful journal. I don't write in it everyday, just here and there. I also like to tape things on the pages that remind me about bright spots in this dark time. My journal has a concert ticket, sweet things my kids say, a handwritten note from a friend, a card from a getaway with my hubby…you get the idea. On my especially

low days, reading through this journal brings me perspective and reminds me that even though I am in a dark place, my life isn't ALL bad.

>>>**Beat the crap out of something.** Yes, I'm for real. You're going to love this, I promise. Early on, I realized that there were some days and some news and emotions that were just too big for me to carry around. Praying, writing in my journal, crying, talking to a friend or Nikita, none of it came close to helping me carry this anger and anguish I was experiencing. I needed a way to release these emotional toxins inside of me. I told Nikita I wanted his help. I asked him to get me an old metal filing cabinet. He looked at me with a look of confusion. "Why?," he asked. I went on to tell him that I wanted an old metal filing cabinet so I could beat the crap out of it with a beat-up metal baseball bat I bought from the Goodwill store for $1.99. A mixture of fear and bewilderment spread across his face, but he said that he would do it. As the weeks went by, I would remind him from time to time and he said he was working on it. Finally one day (once I had forgotten about it), Nikita had me come into our room and there was something really awkwardly wrapped in balloon wrapping paper. I seriously had no clue what he was up to. I opened it and saw a baby blue filing cabinet! I cannot tell you how excited I was. I felt like a kid on Christmas when you get the big gift you asked for. I couldn't wait to take the first swing. Words don't really come close, but let's just say it felt freakin' awesome! It was addicting, too. Once I started hitting it, I just kept going. It felt so good to see and feel the damage my pain was doing to this poor little filing cabinet.

My kids were a little worried about me at first when I would go out to the garage and they could hear the loud banging, but now the cabinet is part of our family culture. Sometimes I'll be at the end of myself (usually around five o'clock in the midst of dinner prep when I'm trying to also help with homework, and deal with the dog following my every move), and I'll just excuse myself, head to the garage, pick up the bat, and get a few swings in before coming back to my crazy reality. Sometimes as I take a whack at the cabinet, I yell out what I've lost, what feels overwhelming, or what I'm grieving. My kids even put on their safety glasses and take a whack at it from time to time. It doesn't change your circumstances, but for a bit, it feels pretty darn good.

I'm not promoting violence here, but there is something to be said for having a physical outlet for your grief. If you were like, "That's awesome," as you read about my filing cabinet, you should definitely get one, or something like it. If that's not your jam, find something else. A punching bag, a kick boxing class, or I've even heard about rage rooms that people can visit to let out their aggressions. Whatever you end up doing, make sure it's a legal and a safe way to unleash your inner Hulk.

Okay friend, you got this. Even though grieving may feeling daunting, exhausting, and scary, please remember that it is your friend. It will be the bridge that leads you to not just accepting your new reality, but eventually embracing the life that lies ahead of you. When you feel weary, look at your Post-it Note on your mirror to remember why you are doing this. You can thank me later.

Chapter 11

PERMISSION

When I was a kid, I always loved going on field trips. It was an opportunity to get out of the classroom and get a break from studying my multiplication tables, doing sustained silent reading, and taking spelling tests. Field trips brought a sense of freedom and adventure, and a chance to see the world from a different perspective. They were a welcome interruption offering a breath of fresh air, and space from the routine and monotony of classroom learning.

One of my favorite field trips was when my fellow sixth graders and I piled into a school bus and headed to Camp Nawakwa for a week of outdoor education. One week out of the classroom with my friends in the great outdoors. It was awesome! We got to take part in all the typical camp fun, like eating crappy cafeteria food, hiking, making crafts, playing pranks on the boys' cabins, hula dancing during Hawaiian night, making up "diddies" to get into dinner, staying up too late in our cabins, and of course, singing around the campfire.

Maybe the best part was just being away from home for a week (sorry, Mom). There was something special about getting out of my routine, breathing in the mountain air, seeing the stars, and making memories with my friends while we still had the freedom to just be kids.

The thing is, none of that would have happened if my parents hadn't done one thing—sign my permission slip. Instead of having one of the best weeks of my twelve-year-old life, if my parents hadn't signed the slip, I probably would have been put into one of the fifth grade classrooms for the week while all of the other sixth graders were gone. I'm not sure that there could be anything more humiliating when you're a big sixth grader than to be left behind with the fifth graders.

Thank you, Mom, for signing that paper. Maybe you and Dad got a little teary letting your baby get on the bus and drive into the mountains to a place you had never been. Or maybe you were high-fiving Margaret Wall, Patti Stolo, and your other mom friends as soon as we were out of sight. Either way, I'm thankful you let me go. I'm thankful you signed the paper and gave me permission to get outside of my small, safe bubble and do something that you knew would be good for me.

So, what does Camp Nawakwa have to do with breast cancer? I'm getting there. During my journey with breast cancer, I told my husband many times, "I just wanna run away." I wished I could run so far and so fast that I could forget about all of the hell I was going through. Bill Murray said it best in the movie *What About Bob?*, "I need a vacation from my problems."

I know you get it. Anyone who has been on a journey like ours needs a vacation. How about a grown up version of Camp Nawakwa? Maybe somewhere tropical, beautiful, and sunny (but not too hot, because of the hot flashes from the estrogen blockade that put my body into early menopause). Actually, anywhere that doesn't involve treatment, doctor visits, or fighting for our lives sounds great. I wish that I could meet you there and we could sip mai tai's and talk about anything but cancer. We could laugh and relax by the pool, and just have a break from this "new normal." Sounds amazing. But heading to Hawaii or Costa Rica in the midst of follow-up doctor's visits, shots, bloodwork, counseling appointments, work, kids' soccer games, homework, and just generally playing catch up from a year of being out of commission, is just not going to happen right now.

Until the time is right to escape to the land where palm trees sway, I want to give you something that has brought a bit of relief to me right where I am. I want to give you something that can be hard to give ourselves—especially if you're a mom. I want to give you permission to give yourself permission. Permission to take a break from this dark season or this depressing day that you feel stuck in. I'm not giving you permission to skip your oncology appointment and run away to Europe indefinitely. Instead, what about permission to do something that makes your burden a little lighter? I want to give you permission to do something to care for yourself today. It might be out of character or something you might not normally make time for, but you know it is exactly what you need; like getting a mani-pedi, not returning text messages, or permission to be creative instead of productive.

This season you are in right now is heavy and hard, and what I'm suggesting won't even come close to tackling what you are facing, but I hope that it would be just a small something to make the burden a little lighter. I hope you can give yourself permission to care for yourself like you would for a friend who is going through a tough time. In fact, as soon as I mentioned this idea, I would venture to guess, you already know exactly what you need right now.

So, here's your mission, should you choose to accept it. Today, and every day until this becomes second nature, I want you to write yourself a permission slip. I don't know exactly what you need permission to do, so you'll have to fill it in yourself. The only advice I'll offer is to make sure it's not something you "should" do, but something that you are allowing yourself to do. Something that would make you laugh or smile, relax, replenish, rest, retreat, or something that makes you feel beautiful when it's hard to look at your bald head in the mirror. Maybe it's even something that releases you from being the "you" that you expect yourself to be, but just can't be right now. It doesn't have to be huge, but something that's just for you—like when I bought myself ranunculus from Trader Joes and picked up my *Magnolia Journal* magazine instead of washing dishes. Or when I told Nikita I didn't have it in me to tell him how my oncology appointment went, and instead I chose to laugh with him at Jimmy Fallon doing, "Thank you notes" on a Friday night.

I will admit that I'm suggesting that you do this, but it does not come easily for me. For some reason, caring for myself feels selfish; I don't know why because I would never call someone else selfish for doing something that breathes life into themselves. I know I'm hard on myself and the standards I have for myself are much higher than anything I would expect of anyone else, but as my counselor would say, there's a difference between selfishness and self-care. Selfishness is only thinking of yourself, what benefits you, and not considering how your actions affect others. I know that's not you, and it's not me. Self-care is just what it sounds like, caring for yourself. And just like all the other human beings you care for, you also deserve to be taken care of. What a novel concept.

Actually, I probably should have had Nikita write this chapter because he is the master of self-care. In fact, he naturally created something that I've affectionately named the "add-on." Let me explain. Let's say there's an errand that needs to be done, like navigating the crowds at Costco on a Saturday. Nikita bravely volunteers and I breathe a sigh of relief. I give him the list and send him on his way. After a couple of hours, I start to wonder where in the world he is. After a few unanswered texts and calls, he calls to tell me he had "added on" coffee with a friend. My initial reaction is annoyance and frustration, but only because he didn't communicate with me what he was up to so I wouldn't expect him sooner. The self-care time with a friend at his favorite coffee shop is actually highly encouraged because I know how refreshed and filled up he is from his time with friends. I call it the "add-on" because he will often add on something for himself when he's out and about doing something for me or the family. Brilliant, right? Me on the other hand, I will just run myself ragged trying to accomplish everything on my list for everyone else, and then by the end of the day, I'm so exhausted I don't have the time or energy to care for myself.

Self-care is a non-negotiable, especially right now. Caring for yourself is what the airline attendants would call, "Putting your own mask on first before assisting others." Self-care is essential because if you don't have your own supply of oxygen, you won't have the ability to be any good for anyone around you. Of course, this makes sense in the midst of an airplane emergency, but it also makes sense now. The reality is, you are in a bit of a crisis yourself. I think it's time to put that mask on. Your body needs oxygen just like everyone else's. It is not selfish to take care of your needs; it is common sense. It is how you will last for the long haul.

Years ago when I read *The 7 Habits of Highly Effective People* by Stephen Covey[1], he wrote about the same concept. He calls it taking time to "Sharpen the Saw." Basically, if you are cutting down a tree with a handsaw, when you sense that you are working harder than you need to be, it's important to sit down and sharpen the saw. His point is that if you take time to sharpen the saw, not only are you getting some much-needed rest, you are also sharpening your saw so that when you start cutting again, you will actually be more effective and finish the job sooner while expending less energy.

Unfortunately, the world doesn't stop just because you are battling cancer. Many people need to continue working, raise kids, make dinner, and clean the house. Hopefully people have stepped up to help with some of these roles in the midst of treatment, but at some point you will need to start assuming responsibilities again even when you are not physically or emotionally functioning at full capacity. Let God use this time as a tool to teach you to care for yourself. It's not practical or wise to just drop everything and run from your oncology follow-ups or unwanted results. However, as you are looking cancer in the face, it's important to not get lost in the hype. Listen to your body and your soul to see what you need. Some days, you may need to give yourself mini vacations to escape, a burst of self-care to renew your body and soul, or time to pause and sharpen the saw in a way that feels refreshing and nurturing. We haven't met yet, but I already know this is what you need. Will you give yourself permission to care for yourself? You're worth it. Below I've listed some things that have been helpful for me, but I would encourage you to make your own list and then start writing those permission slips.

GIVE YOURSELF PERMISSION TO...

SLEEP IN
Set your alarm for an hour later or crawl back in bed once the kids are off to school. Unfortunately, staying in bed all day is not a healthy option on a regular basis, but sometimes an extra hour or two gives your body the boost it needs. Please don't call yourself lazy or shame yourself (like I sometimes do). This battle takes a lot out of you physically and also emotionally, so it's okay to allow yourself to sleep longer than you normally would.

PLAY HOOKY
Take a break from your responsibilities. Go for a walk at the beach, go to the movies in the middle of the day, or call a friend to see if they can meet you for an impromptu coffee date.

GRIEVE
Even though it's hard to go there, it's important to honor what has been lost (review the last chapter) and to wrestle with where you are now.

This is an important part of sharpening the saw in order to prepare you to embrace what is next.

NOT BE PRODUCTIVE
Our society tends to measure the success of a day or of your life by what you've accomplished. When you are going through cancer treatment, this can be problematic because there are times that you just feel stuck and don't have the same capacity or motivation that you had before you went into a tailspin.

It's okay to not always be productive or cross off everything on your to-do list. Those things will still be there tomorrow. You have permission to just be.

PUT YOURSELF IN A TIME-OUT

As a mom, I would seriously love it if someone put me in a time-out. A place where no one is talking to me, touching me, or needing me. It's okay to take a breather instead of pushing through like you used to. My favorite self-imposed time-out is the bathroom. I don't necessarily have to use the bathroom, it's just the only room with a lock so it's the perfect spot to catch my breath and get a five-minute break from whatever is pushing me over the edge.

FIND A GOOD READ

This could be a good book you've been wanting to read or a magazine to catch up on all the latest everything. Whatever you choose, make it something light, fun, or entertaining, with absolutely no mention of cancer.

WATCH SOMETHING THAT MAKES YOU LAUGH

At times it can be difficult to combat the the sad days and heaviness during a cancer journey, so watching something that gives you a deep belly laugh and takes your mind off the hard stuff, can be good for your soul. There are so many good choices...Jimmy Fallon[2], rewatching *Friends*, the silly movie *EuroVision*[3], the stupid pet videos on YouTube, or the latest rom-com. Nikita and I watched *Gilmore Girls*[4] during my treatment, and we found that life in fictitious Stars Hollow was just what we needed. Laughter really is the best medicine.

BE A HOT MESS
You don't have to have it all together, okay? How could you? You're going through it. I'm just proud of you for showering a few times a week and sometimes thinking about shaving your legs.

REMOVE YOURSELF FROM STRESSFUL SITUATIONS
There's nothing like stress to drain the life out of you, and that is the exact opposite of what we are trying to accomplish. You just don't have the emotional bandwidth to deal with this on top of everything else, just remove yourself from the situation. If your kids are arguing over which game to play, ask your husband to sort it out. If your husband wants to talk about the latest political drama (completely hypothetical example), change the subject or ask him to find a friend to hash it out with.

TREAT YOURSELF
Oftentimes, we will do something sweet for a friend, but not for ourselves. Buy yourself fresh flowers from the farmers market or a treat from your favorite ice cream shop. Give yourself a subscription to *Magnolia Journal*, or buy a sweet smelling candle and cozy up. This is the perfect time to start treating yourself again!

LET GO OF A TOXIC RELATIONSHIP
More on this in another chapter, but perhaps your current circumstances can serve as the final push you need to distance yourself from a toxic relationship that has been sucking you dry for way too long. You don't have the extra emotional

energy to spare and even if you did, life is too short for that kind of drama.

NOT TEXT BACK RIGHT AWAY…OR AT ALL.
It's okay. The people that are trying to put themselves in your shoes will understand, and if they're not okay with that, maybe that's the toxic friendship I was referring to above. Your faithful friends will keep texting and ride the wave with you.

MISS YOUR OLD LIFE
At times, it's good to remember life before the cancer turned everything upside down—before you felt scared, and out of control. Don't try to pretend that this life never existed, it's yours and it's an important part of your story. It's okay to miss it and grieve what was lost. I miss my old life, too.

EMBRACE YOUR NEW LIFE
Even though this new life is not what you would have chosen, it's still life. It won't always feel this scary. You will laugh again and go on vacation, and one day people will ask you questions having nothing to do with cancer. You are here and God has a plan and purpose even for this time—embrace it.

ASK FOR WHAT YOU NEED
Even if it inconveniences someone else. People can always say no, but you'll never know if you don't ask. That's how I'm able to write this book. I told Nikita that I felt like God was leading me to write a book about my experience and that I'd need a set time each week to write. He agreed to work from

home on Fridays so that I could have time to get my thoughts down on paper. He is an amazing husband.

NOT COMPARE YOUR JOURNEY TO OTHERS

I've been caught in this trap and trust me, it just never helps. God has written your story just for you. You didn't get cancer because God is out to get you and bless everyone else. But when you compare your life to those around you, it can start to feel that way. Some days will be awful, but other days will be sweet and victorious. Rejoice in your story. It's uniquely yours.

TO ASK SOMEONE NOT TO SAY…

"_____,"

(INSERT INAPPROPRIATE COMMENT ABOUT CANCER HERE)

And then love them anyway.

GET A MANI-PEDI

Having pretty nails always helps me feel beautiful and cared for. Since you're not supposed to do this at the salon during chemo, have a spa night at home. Once chemo is done, head back to the salon to treat yourself.

DO SOME RETAIL THERAPY

No explanation needed. I mean, don't rack up credit card debt, but this is definitely a good time to spend the personal money you've been saving. Go ahead and pamper yourself.

TAKE A DEEP BREATH

Take a deep breath, then let it out, then repeat. If you're like me, the stress of it all causes me to forget to do even the basics, so I end up doing this shallow breathing thing. I feel so much better when taking deep breaths and getting the oxygen my body needs. SoulSpace[5] is a great app that helps you daily engage in relaxing time to slow down your breathing, reflect on a passage from the Bible, and create space to hear from God.

GET MOVING

Exercise is so good for you to clear your head while taking great care of your body. Put on some headphones and listen to some peaceful music or an inspiring podcast while you go for a walk, a hike, or a run. If you are currently going through treatment, be sure to listen to your body and not push yourself too hard. Start slow, you can always increase time or intensity depending on how you are feeling, or what your doctor suggests. I didn't have the same strength or stamina during treatment, but I never regretted getting moving. The point is to care for yourself, so find something that does just that.

GET CREATIVE

Put on some music and draw, do watercolor, or get lost in one of those detailed coloring books. Pick up your guitar that is collecting dust, write poems, build something, or try a new hobby. Find something fun that breathes new life in you.

TELL GOD HOW YOU'RE REALLY DOING

Instead of going through the motions with God or keeping Him at a distance, let Him have it. Hand Him all the burdens you are carrying and share your bitterness, anger, and frustration. He can handle it. Really.

ASK FOR HELP
I know you don't want to, but you need to. Ask a friend or family member to bring dinner or watch your kids so you can go on a date with your hubby or take a nap. No one can read minds, so just ask. People really do want to help, but if they haven't been in your situation, they don't even know what to offer.

NOT LIVE UP TO OTHER PEOPLE'S EXPECTATIONS
You will never make everyone happy, especially not now. This is a great time to use the cancer card. Besides, you are probably barely surviving right now, and they need to be okay with that.

TAKE A NAP IN THE MIDDLE OF THE DAY
I know everything just feels exhausting right now. It's okay to curl up with a cozy blanket and take a thirty-minute break before the kids get home from school.

ASK YOURSELF WHAT YOU NEED
It's always helpful to pause and take stock of what you're feeling today because it'll likely be different than what you needed yesterday…or what you'll need five minutes from now.

TO BE IN PROCESS
Everyone's journey is different, and it's likely that your physical and emotional healing will take longer than you thought. There's no right way to get through this, so there's no point in expecting yourself to be somewhere you're not. You have

permission to be where you are. Take heart, there's still a long way to go, but you're closer than you were yesterday.

TREAT YOURSELF TO SOMETHING SWEET

I know that food cannot solve the deeper ache inside, but some days just call for a sweet treat. Ask a friend to meet you there or have your significant other pick up a pint of your favorite ice cream or the cookie that makes you salivate just thinking about it.

Okay, now it's your turn. Use the permission slip I've provided, or pull out that journal and take some time to brainstorm what you might need in order to care for yourself. I know this won't fix it, but it might help to lighten the load.

SAMPLE PERMISSION SLIP

Due to the storm I've found myself in, I need to care for myself like never before. Tanya told me it's not selfish, it's self-care. Even though I'm used to caring for everyone else first, I'm going to put my needs at the top of the list today because if I don't care for myself, how will I care for those around me?

I, _____ has my permission on
        (FULL NAME)

_____ to _____
  (DATE)   (INSERT SELF CARE IDEA)

        X _____
                (YOUR SIGNATURE)

Chapter 12

BE KIND TO YOURSELF

I remember sitting in my primary care physician's office when I was in the thick of recovery and treatment, and sharing with her my list of questions and concerns over the aches and pains I was feeling physically and emotionally. I was a wreck and I felt like I would never be able to get my act together to function, or even have the capacity to love and care for myself as well as others in my life. It felt like cancer had hijacked my life and I couldn't seem to find my footing. She listened for a while, then she paused, looked at me with much compassion, and gently reminded me to be kind to myself. *Why didn't I think of that?* Immediately the tears started rolling down my face. I didn't realize it, but that was exactly what I needed to hear. That's what I would have said to a friend in my shoes, or to one of the athletes I work with who felt like her world was falling apart. I felt grace washing over me. There is a lot of freedom that comes when you allow yourself to be right where you are, no agenda, no time table, just lots of love and kindness. This season of life is hard enough, there's no room for judgment and criticism.

Even before cancer entered into my story, I've always seemed to have a higher standard for myself than I held for anyone else. I tend to give others the benefit of the doubt, but I am always quick to judge myself. Even though I've grown a lot in this area over the years, my natural tendency is to compare myself to others and I never seem to measure up. In my eyes, it seems like everyone else has it more together than me. I even found myself comparing myself to others who had gone through the cancer journey and wondered why I couldn't have more of a positive outlook or trust God the way they did. It's tough trying to live up to my own standards.

When I was recovering from surgery, and then later going through chemo and radiation, I just didn't have the bandwidth to give, pour out, and kick butt with all of my duties like I had before. For the first time, I really felt my limits and I didn't like it. Suddenly I had to begin to pick and choose what or who I wanted to give my time and energy to that day. I hated it. I wanted to do it all, like I attempted to before, but my body was telling me no, so I had to choose.

As a result, I realized that I had to scale back to do only what was essential. I started with our family. I knew that I wanted my kids and my husband to get the best of me, so often times I would nap about an hour before the kids came home from school so I could give them my best once they were home and Nikita was home for the evening. I also wasn't always able to do the things I normally would do like volunteering in the classroom, helping with homework, driving to soccer practice, hosting playdates, or grocery shopping. My initial reaction was to judge myself and feel like I was slacking. But then as I took a step back, I had to acknowledge the fact that I was entering unchartered water, so I needed to adjust. I told myself I could always add more later if I felt up to it. It was difficult for me to admit that I had limited capacity and energy, but I had to save what I had for the most important things—my inner circle of people. I would remind myself again and again that it was a season, and I wouldn't always be in this place where I had such a small amount to give.

At work, I could have taken a medical leave, but having something to do outside of my home felt like a breath of fresh air. It gave me an opportunity to have a break from my reality and connect with others.

There were times when it made me feel almost normal. However, I knew that even though I wanted things to be business as usual at work, I couldn't serve the way I had before. At work, I decided to give the little time and energy I had to just the female student leaders. It was difficult to limit myself, but being kind to myself meant I needed to know my limits and honor them. In my weaker moments, I would listen to the lie that I was letting my family down or our ministry team down (especially since I was the only female staff person). I would think back to what a typical day was like when I would meet with athletes on campus throughout the day, and then come home and juggle drop offs, pick ups, dinner, and all the other responsibilities that come with managing a household. This was not helpful.

Eventually, I had to surrender what I wanted ministry and my family life to look like. I had to trust God would take care of those athletes I couldn't make time for. I had to believe my husband and kids would feel loved and cared for by the quality time I was able to give them (regardless of the amount), not by me being Super Mom and having the house in perfect order or everything checked off my list. And honestly, the kids don't care who is making their meals or folding their laundry, just as long as the food is good and they have clean undies.

I had to begin to give myself the same grace and compassion I easily extend to others. I was in new territory, so it felt out of control and like I was only a fraction of the woman I used to be. I had to remind myself that I wouldn't be in that place forever, but for now, I needed to care for myself by setting aside my expectations to be everything to everyone. I could still be present and care for these important people in my life, but I had to learn to be okay with the fact that my love for them would look different during this season. God was enough for them and even though I had to pull back, His strength hadn't diminished. He was able to care for me, as well as for those I wanted to care for but couldn't.

I hope that you, too, can extend some extra kindness to yourself, especially during the darkest days. There will be so many times when you'll get to the end of yourself and you won't have anything left in the tank. That's okay. Maybe your kids' hair won't look as cute as when you do it, or maybe the mail will sit unopened longer than usual. And maybe you won't have the strength to care for anyone but yourself today. It's okay. It really is. You have your A-team around you and they will pick up the slack for you when you are just trying to put one foot in front of the next. You won't always be in this place and it won't always be this hard. Be kind to yourself, friend.

Chapter 13

CELEBRATE ALONG THE WAY

"There is a time for everything, and a season for every activity under the heavens." Ecclesiastes 3:1 NIV[1]

Celebration seems like a weird thing to have on your packing list during the middle of this nightmare journey. When I was in the throes of it all, most of the time I was just trying to muster up enough strength to do what I could to care for my family and keep my job. It was honestly a moment-by-moment thing, and it took so much out of me just to find emotional stability to not be a complete basket case 24/7.

Facing cancer is fierce and often times it's a matter of surviving (literally), instead of thriving. However, early on in this journey, I felt God reminding me to celebrate. It was the opposite of what I felt like doing, but I began to wonder what He meant.

Normally I am a person who loves to celebrate. It brings me so much joy to celebrate with others by making a big deal of the milestones and accomplishments in their lives. It doesn't matter if it's a handmade card or searching for the perfect gift, the important thing is my special someone feels seen and celebrated.

I would say that I'm above average at celebrating others and marking the special occasions in their lives, but when it comes to myself, I'd give myself a C-. Passing, yes, but barely. I love being celebrated, but it's harder for me to go all out for myself.

One of the most valuable things I've learned from my walk with cancer is that I am worth celebrating. I don't have to wait for the big things because there is so much to celebrate along the way.

Celebrations give you a reason to look for the bright spots on this otherwise dark and sometimes straight-up depressing journey. At first I thought I would just have a party at the end of all my treatment, but that felt like a lifetime away, and I needed to break this marathon into smaller, more manageable steps that would eventually lead me to the finish line. Just like my kids with a sticker chart, I needed to take time to celebrate and honor myself throughout the journey and acknowledge the grit it was requiring of me each step of the way.

Here are some ways I took time to celebrate in the midst of such a dark and difficult time:

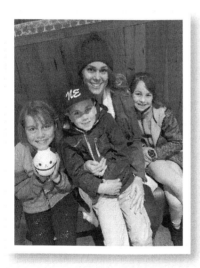

>>> After each chemo infusion, Nikita and I would take a picture with the nurse that was taking care of me that day and then we would head to the beach, try a new restaurant, get a treat, or whatever sounded special and the opposite of what I had just been through. The day of my last chemo infusion, it felt surreal. It was hard to even comprehend that I didn't have to go back again to the infusion room. I could finally exhale...a bit. Nikita and I went to pick up my mom since the kids were still in school and we got fancy doughnuts and coffee at our favorite spot. Later, the kids joined in the fun when we all went for pizza.

>>> Since radiation was six weeks long, I decided that at the end of each week, I would do something fun for myself...try a new dessert spot, get a smoothie, walk around my favorite outdoor mall, buy my favorite candle at Anthropologie (you know the one), or rummage the sale rack at Athleta. Sometimes Nikita was able to join me, but often times, it was just me celebrating me. It felt good to have something to look forward to at the end of each week of radiation.

>>> When I was nearing the end of my third week of radiation, I was thankful to be half way there, but waiting until the end of the six weeks to celebrate felt like an eternity. I needed something to keep me motivated, a goal to work towards so at my halfway point, I decided to bring Krispy Kreme doughnuts and coffee for my amazing radiation oncology team.

>>> March 28, 2019, the last day of radiation, was a BIG day. I couldn't believe I had really reached the finish line. I was so excited to celebrate this HUGE milestone. As I walked through the treatment center door, I was proudly bearing goodies for everyone; monkey bread, Martinelli's sparkling grape juice, notes, and gifts. This was a big day and I was ready to party. What I didn't know was they were planning to celebrate me too. They saw first-hand the perseverance, courage and strength it took to endure this daily battle, and they proudly presented me with a certificate recognizing these attributes. After I got my award, I rang the bell I had been waiting to get my hands on for six weeks; signifying my completion of radiation therapy. I made sure to savor my moment by ringing it

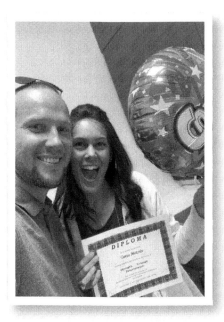

loud and long—it felt liberating! Nikita came in with a balloon and the biggest bear hug. He held me and told me how proud of me he was as tears of joy and relief ran down our cheeks. We took lots of pictures to mark this day and to be reminded of how God had sustained us through it all.

>>> After saying goodbye to my radiation family, Nikita and I went to Huckleberry, one of our special occasion breakfast spots, and I savored every bite. This meal signified the completion of months of blood, sweat, and tears. At times I thought that I'd never make it to this moment, yet there I was.

>>> A few weeks later, we invited our friends, family, my doctors, and our neighbors to come and enjoy street tacos and dessert as we celebrated the fact that I was done with treatment and cancer was behind me. It was a magical evening for me, as I was surrounded by dear ones who had prayed for me, served me, encouraged me, cried with me, and stuck with me through my dark night of the soul. Even some of the men from Nikita's men's prayer group, who I had never met but who had been praying for me throughout the year, were there to help us celebrate. It was amazing.

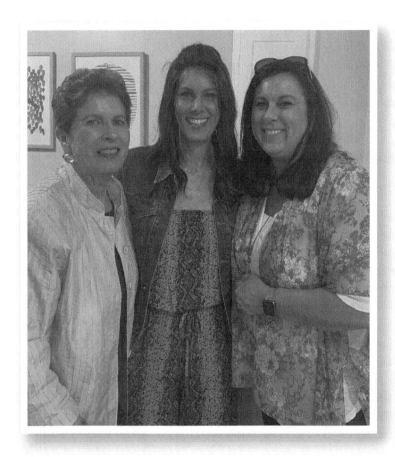

>>> Weeks before the celebration I had told Nikita that I wanted him to get me some kind of trophy or medal to commemorate what I had been through. Like my kids get medals at the end of their soccer seasons, or when I received my diplomas from Pepperdine, I felt that I had earned something special for what I had accomplished. I had kind of forgotten about mentioning this to Nikita, but he hadn't. During the celebration, our friends and family gathered together so we could share a few words and many tears. I remember looking around at each face in the crowd and my heart felt so full.

We thanked everyone for the part they had played in getting us through that year, and of course we thanked God for the beautiful ways He had loved us and strengthened us through each of the people looking back at us. It was a moment I will never forget.

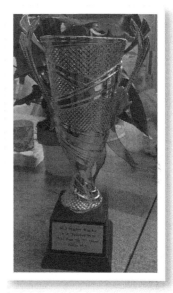

That would have been enough to seal the deal on an unforgettable night for me, but then Nikita began to share with our guests how I had asked him to get me a trophy or a medal to commemorate all I had been through. With that, everyone started laughing. But instead of laughter, I had tears of joy when he pulled out a shiny, plastic, beautiful trophy. I felt like the warrior that I was as I held my champion's cup and read the inscription that made me catch my breath, "To a mighty warrior. To my wife who beat the c word. Psalm 46:5²." It wasn't just a trophy to me, it represented so much more, and there are many more words that could never fit on the inscription. It was perfect. This year wouldn't have been complete without this time to celebrate.

>>> After completing my treatment our family decided to spend a few nights away on Catalina Island. This was such a special time to explore the island, go for a hike, grill on the balcony overlooking the ocean, and acknowledge that we had all done this together.

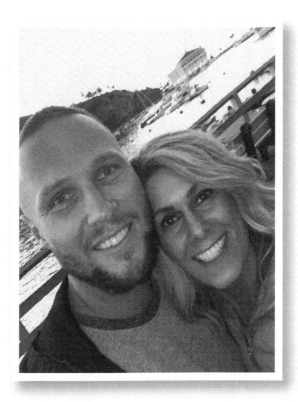

I hope that you, too, can find some special ways to celebrate along the way. Maybe sharing my celebrations will give you some ideas. You know what you need more than anyone, so perhaps instead of a big party, it's a small intimate gathering; whatever feels celebratory to you. The important thing is to celebrate. We know better than most that we are not guaranteed tomorrow, so take time to celebrate the bright spots on this dark road. You've earned it.

PART 3
Getting Down To Business

Chapter 14

BREAST SURGEON: DECIDING ON WHICH SURGERY

As soon as I found out there was cancer in my body, I wanted it out yesterday. Unfortunately, the conversations that need to be had and the decisions that need to be made can feel like obstacles keeping you from getting it out, but they are important for your future well-being.

When I first met my breast surgeon, I could tell right away she was brilliant and really knew her stuff. Clearly, there was a reason she was the head of the Revlon Breast Center at UCLA. She shared with me that she herself had gone through breast cancer and had undergone a double mastectomy. Even though the thought of a double mastectomy scared me to death, I was so thankful to be in the hands of someone who was not only one of the best in her field, but someone who really understood what it was like to be in my shoes. That was priceless.

As I spoke with my doctor, there was still part of me that hoped she would examine me, do all the scans, and come back to tell me there was no cancer. Accepting life-altering news has a way of catapulting you into an alternate reality that can take months to accept. It's shocking news you weren't expecting, so it takes time to allow it all to sink in. I was completely overwhelmed as we met together. I could hear the words coming out of her mouth, but it was difficult to take everything in.

"Lumpectomy, stage one, mastectomy, Tamoxophen, nipple-sparing," it all felt like a foreign language to me. I asked her about the lumpectomy, but she felt that a lumpectomy wasn't a good option due to the size of my breasts. There just wasn't enough breast tissue. This was a blow not only because she was saying my boob was too small to take the cancer out and still have a normal boob left, but also because that only left me with the option of mastectomy. This felt like a crappy option.

Even though I didn't have any cancer in my left breast, now I had to decide if I should go ahead and have a bi-lateral mastectomy. Even though my doctor didn't say I needed to, I didn't know if I wanted to have one boob with an implant (a tiny one apparently) and one without.

This felt like a huge decision for me because I didn't want to have a bi-lateral mastectomy if I didn't have to. I mean my left boob was perfectly healthy and there was no sign of cancer. Thank God. There were other women I had gotten in touch with who had similar situations and some decided to have a single mastectomy and others went for the double. But for me, there was this nagging fear in me wondering if the cancer would spread or come back one day in my other breast. I also learned that my chances of getting cancer in my left breast were higher once I had it in my other breast. Some of the breast cancer survivors I spoke with said that for them, they didn't want to remove a perfectly good breast and that if it came back one day, they would go through the surgery again. After all, they had done it once, they knew they could do it again. But for me, the thought of waiting and wondering if it would show up in my other breast was too much to consider. I didn't think I could be at peace about leaving my left breast untouched. I was heavily leaning towards doing the double, but I decided to schedule another appointment with my doctor so I could ask all the questions that I didn't think to ask the first time. I wanted to be sure that I wasn't making my trauma even more traumatic by removing both breasts instead of just one. When

I was trying to decide what to do, I remember talking to my friend, Melinda (a fellow breast cancer survivor), about it and her insight helped me. She said that even if I decided to just do the single, it wouldn't be any less traumatic. Either way my body would never be the same. My scars and missing nipple on one side would always remind me that a wrecking ball had come through.

In the end, I didn't want to look back one day and wish I had done the double. I didn't want to regret the fact that I hadn't done all that I could to prevent this monster from rearing it's ugly head again. I was going to be traumatized either way, so I decided to go with the more cautious route and do the double.

As you look at your options and weigh all of the pros and cons, try to remember a couple of things. First, this is YOUR body. If your doctor has given you a choice, you need to pray, ask your doctor lots of questions, and talk to as many breast cancer survivors as you can to see why they made the decision they did. Also, keep in mind that all of the people you turn to are simply consultants helping you to make the best possible decision for YOU. This is your body and, at the end of the day, you are the one who will need to live with your decision. So, once you've prayed (or "trusted your gut" as some women told me) and gathered up all of the input and experience from others, make the decision that feels best for you, and then don't look back.

Chapter 15

PLASTIC SURGEON: DECIDING ON WHICH SURGERY

After I met with my breast surgeon for the first time, her assistant worked her magic and got me in that day to meet with the Chief of Plastic Surgery for UCLA. As Nikita and I were making our way over to the next building, my head was still spinning from all my doctor had told me. Now I needed to shift gears and think about the cosmetic side of things.

Before I met my plastic surgeon, I figured I had two options: implants or no implants. I was thankful to be in the hands of an expert who gave me a third option. I was so impressed with my plastic surgeon's bedside manner, knowledge, patience, and understanding. He even made me laugh at one point (a rare thing during this scary time for me). He was very thorough, asked good questions about what I wanted (and Nikita chimed in, too), and then he began to tell me my different options. One breast, two breasts, implants, no implants, and then he told me about something I had never heard of—DIEP flap reconstruction. Basically, DIEP flap reconstruction is when the breast surgeon does a single or double mastectomy (whatever you've decided) to remove all the cancer and breast tissue, then the plastic surgeon makes a lower abdominal incision (think same area as a C-section, but longer, like hip to hip) and removes belly tissue to reconstruct your breast(s).

From the get-go, the DIEP flap reconstruction intrigued me. Initially my doctor wasn't sure that I'd have enough fat to form two breasts (thank you Weight Watchers), but leave it to the plastic surgeon, after yanking on my belly a bit, he concluded that there would be enough tissue to construct two small breasts. I was worried though about the "small breast" part. I mean, my breasts were already really small, so I asked him if they could turn out even smaller. He said no, they would be about the same size or maybe even a bit bigger. Okay, that seemed reasonable.

I think I was curious about this option partially because it was a choice I didn't know existed and, at a time when so much was out of my control, it felt good to have some kind of say in the matter. I also liked the fact that my own tissue would be used to reconstruct my breasts instead of using implants. Don't get me wrong, implants are a very good option, but I've always been a bit of a "tree hugger" as my dad would call me, so the idea of a natural option and not having to worry about leaks or replacing implants down the road, really appealed to me. The part that didn't sound so good was the nine hours (or more) in surgery, the longer recovery in the hospital (five days vs. one day), the scar stretching from hip to hip, and the longer recovery at home (no sleeping on my stomach or side for twelve weeks!). On top of all this, being a people pleaser made this decision a hard one. I wanted to get implants to please Nikita, I mean why not take the opportunity to go up a cup size (or two)? I also wanted to take the least amount of risk, so the shorter surgery and shorter recovery seemed to be the "wisest" choice for a mom with three young kids. However, I also needed to go with what I felt most comfortable with since it was my body. After praying a lot, talking to friends, and friends of friends who had different breast surgeries, and having what felt like a million conversations with Nikita where he assured me that he would love my boobs no matter what size they were, I decided to go with the DIEP flap reconstruction. At the end of the day, I had to go with what felt right to me, because it was my body, and I was the one who would have to live with my decision. It also felt good to know that Nikita was supporting me either way. Once I finally made my decision, I had so much peace. I had such a sense of relief now that I had that major decision behind me and I was one step closer to recovery. I had to laugh too that within my first two months of being back in LA, I was already assimilating well into the culture by getting a boob job and a tummy tuck. Hollywood, here I come.

Chapter 16

GENETIC TESTING

Genetic testing was an aspect of my cancer journey I wasn't expecting. Chances are, before surgery, you will undergo genetic testing to give your team of doctors a better picture of your unique situation.

The same day that I met with my doctors, (and signed our rental agreement for a place to live), I walked over to get my blood drawn for genetic testing and to meet with the genetic counselor. I felt overwhelmed by all her questions about my health history, like when I started my period or if anyone in my family had a history of breast or ovarian cancer. Some of the questions made sense, but others were difficult for me to connect to breast cancer. It was helpful when the counselor shared with me that there are different factors that they look at to determine if you are at a higher risk for developing breast cancer.

The counselor also explained to me that they would be testing my genetic make up in two layers. First they look at a group of eight genes which are the most common genes linked to breast cancer. Included in that group are the BRCA1 and BRCA2 genes. We would get the results back from the group of genes most connected to breast cancer first, and then they would test for a larger group of genes loosely connected to breast cancer.

After getting all the genetic testing done, I found out a couple weeks later that everything came back negative, which brought a huge wave of relief, but also confusion. I wondered, *If I don't have the "cancer genes" and none of the other risk factors apply to me, why do I have breast cancer?* It didn't make sense.

Regardless of why you have breast cancer, it's not what you were planning on. It doesn't make sense and it's not fair. Unfortunately, life has so many loose ends and there are no formulas that lead to guaranteed good health. There are things that we can do to avoid or lower our risk of walking into a health landmine (more on this in a later chapter), but there are no guarantees. This reality is still hard for me to accept. I wish I could tell you otherwise.

COVERED

CaringBridge Journal entry by Tanya Motorin
September 30, 2018

Thank you all for your thoughts and prayers over the past few days. It's hard to believe that I'm already heading into my last night at the hospital and they are prepping me for my discharge tomorrow.

When I was preparing for surgery earlier this week, I had asked different people to ask the Lord for a specific word or verse for me as I headed into Wednesday. I was so encouraged to hear from the Lord in that way. Some words and verses shared with me were... Whole, "I love you," promises from Isaiah 43-1:4[1], faithful, prisoner of hope, honored, fear of the Lord leads to life, Rock.

The morning of my surgery I woke with a feeling of "let's do this" mixed with an overwhelming feeling of dread. I also realized that I needed to ask the Lord for a specific word or phrase for me. I wanted to hear directly from Him. As soon as I asked, I heard the word, "Covered." I knew exactly what He meant. And it was perfectly what I needed to be reassured of.

COVERED. Like the Israelites who were leaving what they knew and heading toward a new land. They were led by the fire at night and covered by the cloud during the heat of the day.

COVERED. By so many of you who have already stepped up to cover our family with meals and gift cards, additional ministry support, watching our kids, finding and delivering a recliner for post-surgery recovery, and even cold hard cash to help cover the growing medical bills.

COVERED. As in Psalm 91:4[2] He will cover you with His feathers. He will shelter you with His wings. His faithful promises are your armor and protection.

COVERED. Like my kids that want to be cozy warm as I tuck them in at night and later that night when I make sure their blanket is still covering them before I head to bed.

COVERED. I needed to know that He wasn't just with me, but that He was a part of me... like my skin. Covering me.

When I woke up from surgery 9.5 hrs later, the first thing I felt was relief. The one who created me and knows my body better than any doctor, had me COVERED.

Chapter 17

STEPPING INTO BATTLE

There's a reason why people say that they are "battling cancer." Facing cancer is not for the faint of heart. You need your armor to be victorious. For me, the armor wasn't heavy or made of metal. My armor was comprised of the prayers of many warriors that were stepping into battle with me. And even though I felt sick to my stomach, I knew that I was covered, not only by the prayers of so many, but by the promises of my faithful God. I didn't like that He was allowing me to go through this, but if I had to walk this path, I knew I needed His covering.

Nikita and I headed to the hospital at some ungodly hour that morning, and I felt scared, but peaceful at the same time. It felt scary to face this giant, but this step in the battle was an important one; I would finally be cancer free.

When Nikita dropped me off at the hospital roundabout, I was welcomed by Keenan, my close friend over the last twenty years. I was in Jen and Keenan's wedding, they were in ours, and he has since become a dear friend to Nikita as well. Keenan brings the perfect mix of inside jokes, laughter, and empathy. He is not only a friend, but also a pastor. His presence calmed me, but also brought me to tears. I didn't know he was going to be there, but I think God knew that we both needed some extra support and encouragement as we stepped into the ring with cancer. As we sat in the waiting room it was probably annoying to those around us as I told him about having to stop for an unexpected poop at the gas station before arriving to the hospital that morning. The three of us were bent over laughing. Laughter was the last thing I thought I would be doing in the waiting room, but it was also good to have a diversion and someone to chit chat with so I didn't have to think as much about what was waiting for me upstairs.

Eventually the nurse came to get me, and Keenan came with us upstairs to pray for us before he left. I needed that too. After he left, the nurse came to give me some instructions and told me to strip down and put on my gown. While I was in the restroom I got another surprise. Out of 365 days in a year, my body decided to start my period on the one day I was heading into surgery. Perfect. Now I had to put on those fishnet undies with a huge pad stuck inside. Good times. I guess it's not uncommon for you to start your period during times of stress, but I think my period just wanted to make a special appearance before my body was forced into menopause. Either way, it wasn't what I was dreaming of.

After that I was back in my makeshift room when Dr. Chang, my breast surgeon, and then Dr. DaLio, my plastic surgeon, came to check in with me. It was good to see some familiar faces, but I wished they were there to check on me after surgery instead of having surgery still in front of me. They were both all business, which I guess you want on the morning of your surgery. Instead of comfort and hand holding, I want surgeons with their game faces on and ready to live up to their outstanding reputations.

After they left, there was more waiting. I took a good look at my faithful husband who had driven me there, got me to a restroom in time, and held my hand throughout the morning, and God reminded me that I had chosen well. In sickness and in health. This was our chance to live out our vows, to show the world around us that what God brings together, no man can separate. We prayed one more time just the two of us and then came the hardest part...letting go of his hand as the nurse came in to wheel me into the main operating room. I prayed one more silent prayer that this wouldn't be the last time I looked into his soft blue eyes.

Nine and a half hours later, they were done with surgery. I remember waking up for the first time and being so thankful that I was alive and that I had made it through surgery. The cancer was gone, and I had two new (very sore) boobs! So much to be thankful for! Thank You, Jesus.

After five days in the hospital, I was more than ready to get home, but I also felt nervous about heading back into my world and wondering if I would have what it took to be the warrior I knew I needed to be.

If you haven't had your surgery yet, I know that the thought of surgery feels scary, but it's the first step that will get you closer to the end of this journey. You got this. You are braver than you think.

Here are some things to remember as you prepare for surgery:

When you are packing your bag, remember to include a post-mastectomy bra to wear while you are recovering. My doctor recommended the pink Elizabeth-brand post-mastectomy bra which was super. It is so soft and comfortable and it even has rings on it that you can attach your post-surgery drains to. I ended up getting two so I could have one on while I was washing the other one. If I remember correctly, one was covered by my insurance. If your hospital doesn't have a cancer boutique with bras and other essentials, be sure to ask the staff at your doctor's office or other breast cancer survivors you know, where you can find the items you need for recovery.

Also be sure to pack some really loose fitting comfortable pants (if you're having the DIEP flap surgery), and a button-up or loose fitting shirt that you can get on without raising your arms. A friend of mine also gave me some small pillows to put under the seat belt so I didn't have any rubbing or chaffing while I was in the car. These were life- savers and I used them for weeks after the surgery.

In addition to the essentials, I also brought some magazines, a book, and my journal. I don't know if I thought I was going on a weekend retreat instead of going in for major surgery, but needless to say, I didn't get any reading done. What I did end up looking at a lot, were the pictures of friends and family as well as a favorite Bible passage that I had asked Nikita to put on the wall across from my bed. Having that wall covered with those I love most was so encouraging whenever I came in and out of sleeping. As I looked at the wall, I was quickly reminded that I was not alone. There were so many people battling cancer with me.

PART 4
Necessary Evils & Disappointing News

Chapter 18

WAITING FOR RESULTS

Once I was home, my world was filled with changing bandages, emptying the drains (two for my boobs and two for my tummy), and sleeping in a recliner for twelve weeks so I wouldn't roll onto my side in the middle of the night. I was glad to be on the road to recovery, but it was most definitely a painful and exhausting one.

It also felt like torture as I waited to hear back from my doctor about the pathology results. I tried not to be consumed by it, but like a boomerang, all the what if's kept returning to me. When she finally called, I rushed into the back room to have a quiet space to hang on her words. My next heartbeat felt suspended mid-beat when she told me that there was a 2.2 millimeter mass in one of the three sentinel lymph nodes they had removed. She went on to say that she wanted me to get a bone scan and chest x-ray to see if anything had spread beyond the lymph nodes. I was devastated. I had been praying so hard that the cancer would be contained to the breast. I knew this meant that radiation wouldn't be enough. My lungs seemed to press down, keeping me from getting a full breath. I wanted to scream or hit something. Or both. This was starting to feel scary again.

A week or so later, I was back at my doctor's office for an interdisciplinary meeting she had set up with the oncologist, radiation oncologist, and the psychologist to meet and discuss my case. After they all met, I met with each of them to hear their recommendations. The radiation oncologist said even though I was kind of in a gray area, he recommended six weeks of radiation therapy, the oncologist said she recommended four rounds of chemotherapy with three weeks in between, and the psychologist, just listened, asked good questions, and gave me some space to grieve the tornado that had just touched down.

The day was a whirlwind, but it was also really helpful to have all the specialists in one place to discuss my case and then decide collectively what they felt the best course of action should be. Even though I was overwhelmed beyond words, I knew I was in good hands. There was a plan and I was preparing for the next battle ahead of me.

Though surgery and treatments are painful, waiting for results can feel excruciating. It can be emotionally exhausting as you try to think through and imagine all of the different scenarios playing out. As you wait, remember that God has purpose in this time as well. It isn't a holding cell He has you in before you head into battle. This is a time to lean into Him and those He has gathered around you on this journey.

This time of waiting prepares you for what is coming next. Take some time to reread Joshua 1:1-9[1]. Prior to this passage, God had raised up Moses to lead the Israelites out of Egypt and into the land He had promised them. However, the journey was longer than they expected and they ended up in the desert for forty years. We pick up the story when Moses had just died and now Joshua was chosen by God to lead the Israelites into the promised land. Right before they cross the Jordan River into the land that God had promised them forty long years before, God gives Joshua a bit of a pep talk. This passage is rich with reminders, promises, and commands from God, but the phrase that sticks with me most is, "Be strong and courageous." God doesn't just say it once, but three times. One of those times He emphasizes and says, "Be strong and very courageous." God knew that just because they were heading into this beautiful land that He had promised them, it wouldn't be all rainbows and sunshine. Joshua and God's people would need to hold on to His command to be strong and courageous. But God doesn't just give Joshua and His people this command as a way to fire them up as they head into another unknown. In verse five, right before God first tells Joshua to be strong and courageous, He reminds them of the source of their strength and courage. God says, "As I was with Moses, so I will be with you…" His presence is what enabled them to be strong and courageous as they stepped into what God had next for them.

The same is true for you. God isn't just telling you to muster up all *your* strength and courage for the battle ahead. He is gently and lovingly reminding you that *He* is your strength and courage. You are not alone.

So, as you wait, take advantage of this space, this time to pause and reacquaint yourself with the God that will never leave you or forsake you. Marinate on this truth. Let it soak into the marrow of your bones in this time of waiting. I know what is coming next doesn't exactly feel like you are stepping into the promised land, but being anchored in His presence, no matter what is coming next, will be the very thing that strengthens you for what lies ahead.

Chapter 19

INCIDENTAL FINDINGS

Reluctantly, I went for the additional scans my doctor wanted me to get, and I was praying that my bone scan and chest CT would come back clear. The bone scan looked good, but the CT showed that I had some nodules in my lung that they wanted to keep an eye on. It also showed something unusual in my left lung. The Pulmonologist I was referred to had me go in for multiple Pulmonary Function tests, and another CT scan. After several weeks, he determined that the nodules were actually scar tissue and the unusual mass in my lung was a cluster of cysts that was determined to be a congenital malformation. Thank God.

In the midst of all the scans and tests, the Pulmonologist also did a full metabolic blood panel and discovered that I had a couple different antibody levels that were higher than normal. I had no idea what that even meant. What I did know was that I was growing weary. These findings led me to more appointments, tests, scans, and monitoring. Instead of moving toward some kind of control or light at the end of the tunnel, I felt like my health was a ball of yarn unraveling as it rolled down hill. One day I was seemingly "healthy" and then I wasn't. With each new specialist, and new scan or test, another "incidental finding" popped up. Just when I could almost come to terms with the latest news or step in the journey, something new would appear and knock me down again physically and spiritually. How much could one woman take? I had already killed so many trees with my countless mile-long CVS drugstore receipts. How could I possibly navigate one more surprise?

I was hesitant to share this with you because the last thing you need is something else to obsess over or worry about. So, please don't. And just because the doctors found other non-cancer related heath issues in my body doesn't mean that will happen to you. Everyone's path is different. Hopefully your story doesn't lead to more medical rabbit trails like mine that, on top of a breast cancer diagnosis, can feel larger than life. It may be health issues or it may be life issues. Work piling up, kids melting down, cars needing repairs, bills that never stop, or someone you love dealing with their own health issues. Unfortunately life doesn't stop just because your world is crumbling. It's a lot to hold. Try to take one day at a time. Matthew 6 is a great one to reread right about now.

"Look at the birds of the air; they do not sow or reap or store away in barns, and yet your heavenly Father feeds them. Are you not much more valuable than they? Can any one of you by worrying add a single hour to your life?" Matthew 6:26-27[1]

God is with you in the mess; today and tomorrow.

Chapter 20
ONCOLOGY

Out of all your doctors, your oncologist is the one you'll be spending the most time with down over the long haul. When considering which oncologist to go with, be sure to find someone that is not only qualified, but someone whom you feel cares about you beyond just eradicating the cancer in your body. Your oncologist isn't your counselor, but in my opinion, he or she needs to acknowledge and affirm the fact that cancer isn't just a lump they remove or cells they treat with medicine or radiation. He or she needs to support the fact that breast cancer is so much more than just dealing with rebellious cells that have mutated. You are a person who has plans, dreams, a family, and fears. Cancer affects all of you.

There were so many times when I was a hot mess as I sat in my oncologist's office, sharing my fears, my aches and pains, and even crying about how three of my friends just died from cancer in the past two months. We locked eyes and I knew she saw my pain as she took time to listen and affirm all that I carried into the office that day. As you search for an oncologist, find someone who not only sees your cancer, but sees you.

Even though I felt comfortable with my doctor and felt seen by her, I had so much anxiety every time I had to go to her office. At first I wondered if I had chosen wisely. I wondered if God was trying to tell me to find somebody different to treat my cancer. After praying about it and talking it over with Nikita, I realized I just didn't like going to the oncologist. I could have had Mother Theresa for a doctor, full of a beautiful display of love and compassion, but I am confident I still would have had that same pit in my stomach even at the thought of going to her office. I hated the fact that I needed an oncologist, and every time I had to see her or think about seeing her, it jolted me back into reality and triggered all the pain and trauma I had already been through.

The first few times I met with my oncologist, I was just trying to keep up with all the information she was sharing about my type of cancer. My biopsy showed that I had invasive ductal carcinoma that was positive for estrogen and progesterone receptors (ER/PR+) and negative for the Her2 protein. My oncologist suggested that we also send my tumor out to a lab to have a MammaPrint test done to determine my tumor's genetic makeup. Having a better understanding of the biology of your tumor can allow you and your doctor to make a more educated decision about which type of treatment you will need.

Since my MammaPrint results showed that my cancer would respond well to chemo, my doctor told me I would need four infusions of Cytoxin and Taxotere every three weeks. After chemo, I would take Letrozole (an aromatase inhibitor), daily for five to ten years. This medication helps to suppress the estrogen that the rest of your body (not just your ovaries) produces. Since I wasn't menopausal, she also recommended Lupron, which is a monthly shot to suppress the estrogen my ovaries were producing.

Obviously your plan will be customized to your tumor markers and genomic testing, but I wanted to share my plan with you, so you have a general idea of what to expect or what to ask your doctor.

As you head into these conversations with your oncologist, be extra kind to yourself before and after those appointments. It was helpful for me to invite my husband and a handful of trusted friends into this space with me, and ask them to be interceding for me before, during, and after these appointments. It still felt scary, but it was reassuring knowing I wasn't facing these appointments alone.

One thing that also helped me as I prepared myself for the oncologist appointments, was to think through questions I had for my doctor ahead of time. This may sound like a no-brainer, but it's important.

Once I'm in the doctor's office, I tend to freeze up and forget to ask the important questions I've been carrying around for the past several weeks. I found it helpful to make a checklist on my phone ahead of time so I felt a bit more in control and I knew what my objectives were heading into my appointment.

Here are some questions you may want to ask your doctor if you haven't already:

- What type of cancer do I have?
- What are my markers?
- Can a MammaPrint test be done on my tumor to determine its genetic makeup?
- Does my insurance cover genomic testing?
- What stage is my cancer?
- Will I need chemotherapy? If so, which kind and for how long? Will it cause me to lose your hair?
- What are the other side affects of this type of chemo?

- Why did you choose this type of chemo?
- Are there certain foods or activities I should avoid while going through cancer treatment?
- Will I need to take medication once I'm done with chemo? If so, which kind and for how long?
- Will I also need radiation therapy?

CHEESE ENCHILADAS

CaringBridge Journal entry by Tanya Motorin
Nov. 19, 2018

So I've never been super great at remembering a ton of details from my childhood, but there is one memory that will never leave me. I was around 12 years old, and my friend Stacy was over for a playdate (although that's not what they were called back then...I'm dating myself now). I'm sure we were having a great time, I wish I could tell you what we were doing (like I said, not all the details have stayed with me), but the part I do remember is my mom having to leave for a bit to run a quick errand. Before she left, she reminded me to eat something for lunch. Stacy had already eaten lunch at home, and I wasn't hungry yet, so the minute she left we went back to playing, whatever it was we were playing. Before we knew it, it was almost time for my mom to return and I suddenly remembered that I was supposed to eat before she got back, so I went to the kitchen to see what my options were. I decided that I wanted one of the frozen meals, so I turned the oven on to allow time for it to preheat. It didn't take long for us to notice a yummy smell coming from the oven. I was thrown off because I hadn't put any food in the oven yet, but when I opened it up, there was a tray with VanDeKamp cheese enchiladas. At first we were confused, but then I drew the conclusion that my mom must have put them in there for me. Cool, I waited a few more minutes and then pulled the enchiladas out and ate them.

My mom came home about 10 min later and the first thing she asked was whether or not I had eaten lunch. "Yep, I ate the enchiladas you put in the oven for me." In complete shock and confusion, she quickly told me that she hadn't put any enchiladas in the oven. Okay, now I was really confused and my mom was growing concerned because she didn't know how long the enchiladas had been in there. After lots of questions and trying to piece together all the parts, we realized that the enchiladas I ate were the same enchiladas my sister had put in the oven the week before while we were having a family reunion at our house. She had to leave early for a soccer tournament, and somehow forgot about the enchiladas until I found them a week later and ate them.

So, my mom, being the great mom that she is, called Dr. Hall's office to see what she should do. After talking to Darlene, the nurse, she ran to Sav-on to pick up a prescription for Ipecac. For those of you who don't know, Ipecac is a medicine that induces vomiting in case of possible poisoning. Ugh. When she got back I had to take the medicine (which seriously tasted like throw up) and then the directions said that in 15 minutes I would begin vomiting. So, Stacy and I continued to play until 15 minutes was up and I went to sit on the floor of our guest bathroom, waiting to throw up. When I started feeling nauseous, I closed the door, did my business, and then the playdate picked up where we left off.

Wow, out of all the childhood memories, this is the one that is forever etched in my mind? Gross. But for some reason, when God brought this memory to mind today, there were tears in my eyes. I guess I can relate to that 12-year-old girl who was waiting to get sick... I, too, am getting ready to take some medicine that will not only make me sick, but will cause me to lose my hair, experience bone pain, tingling in my hands and feet, dry skin, hot flashes...and a whole gamut of other fun side effects. And I'll be honest with you, I am NOT looking forward to any of this. In fact, if I'm really honest, I'm still kind of angry with God and sad that my old life is gone. Grieving has become part of my new normal and even though I haven't even started chemo yet, I already feel exhausted and broken just thinking about it.

So, I know it wasn't a coincidence that God brought this memory to mind for me today (the day before I start chemo). And what He reminded me of specifically was how that little girl handled the side effects coming her way. My 12-year-old self played and enjoyed her friend right up until the medicine started doing its thing. She didn't overanalyze everything, she didn't waste time blaming her sister for leaving the enchiladas in the oven, or blaming herself for eating enchiladas that appeared out of nowhere. She didn't waste her play time worrying about how awful it was going to be to throw up in front of her friend, and she certainly didn't question God's love for her. Maybe she was scared, I mean who likes throwing up? But instead of being stuck in that fear, she did what she was told and as soon as she was done (well maybe after she brushed her teeth), she went back to enjoying her friend.

I know that eating some old enchiladas and having to throw them up is really different than the journey I'm on now. But, what hasn't changed, is Him. God allowed me to endure some momentary discomfort so that the potential poison would not do greater damage. And even though the situations are different, He is the same. He is still the God who has the power to intervene, but sometimes chooses for us to endure some pain and suffering so that we can see the same result that James talks about in the Bible.

Consider it pure joy my brothers and sisters, whenever you face trials of many kinds. Because you know that the testing of your faith produces perseverance. Let perseverance finish its work, so that you may be mature and complete, not lacking anything.

James 1:2-4[1]

You see, I have been so busy dreading chemo, that I've been tempted to take my eyes off of Him. To question His love and plan for me. And today He gently reminded me that His love and His character do not change based on my circumstances. And even though I still hate this, I can also see more clearly that God is actually allowing me to endure chemo because He is good and He wants me to be mature and complete...and to enjoy Him and the life that He has blessed me with. Yes, chemo will bring some terrible side effects, but I'm thankful that God is allowing chemo to also do what it was created to do...keep the cancer from coming back. And that's a good thing.

Chapter 21

CHEMO

Finding out I needed chemo was *not* the news I had been praying for. Not only did I not want toxins pumped into my body, but I was also devastated about the thought of losing my hair. I didn't understand why God continued to lead me down the harder path.

If you are also facing chemo, I'm so sorry. It's this terrible thing that you would never want to go through, and yet, it's the one thing that you need in order to survive. A necessary evil.

CHEMO PREP WORK

It's important to prepare yourself mentally, physically, and spiritually before each infusion.

What I did:

- Painted my nails, spent time with family, prayed with Nikita, packed my bag of essentials so I didn't have to scramble in the morning, and I tried to head to bed earlier than normal

What your doctor may have you do:

- Start taking Claritin a couple days beforehand to help with the nausea
- Take your prescribed steroids the day before

SUGGESTED CHEMO CHECKLIST

(This is just to give you an idea of things that may be helpful to bring with you the day of your infusion, but find what works for you)

- BEAUTY: To keep my skin hydrated under my regular makeup, I used *Innovative Skincare* (a clinical, professional skincare line I was introduced to at UCLA. More on this in Chapter 25). Burts Bees tinted lip balm kept my lips moisturized and the pop of color was my attempt at brightening a dark time. I also brought regular my chapstick in case my lips got dry and hand sanitizer to make sure I was avoiding germs as much as possible.

- COMFORT: I brought a neck pillow and regular pillow from home. For each infusion, I also cozied up with different blankets that friends had sent me.

- ENTERTAINMENT: Magazine, Book, Bible, iPad. It was nice to have options to read, but mostly I was pretty wiped, so I usually just talked with Nikita, read a bit, and then slept.

- CHEMO JOURNAL: It was helpful for me to have a place to track my weight, what I ate, medicines or supplements I was taking, and how I felt physically and emotionally.

- FOOD: For some, chemo can cause a strong metallic taste. It wasn't the case for me, but a friend of mine swears by ginger candies to help with this. Drink plenty of water, your favorite snacks, or whatever sounds good that day.

- TECH: Headphones, phone, phone charger.

- PRACTICAL: Insurance card and ID. Gloves, ice, and cooler (more on this below).

DAY OF: WHAT TO EXPECT

I had to do four cycles of Cytoxan and Taxotere infusions, three weeks apart. It felt scary and required so much courage each time I went. It's important to determine who you might need by your side the day of.

Some people have a different friend or family member come with them to their infusions. For me, I just wanted Nikita there. It already felt like such a vulnerable place to be in. I just wanted him there to steady me and know what I needed instead of having to "train" someone new each time. You'll find what works best for you.

The morning of, I would suggest getting out and moving a bit before you need to go and sit for several hours. I centered my heart and mind on a morning walk and then enjoyed some oatmeal with fruit and nuts and a big glass of water. <u>It's so important to be drinking lots of water</u> before, during, and after the infusion.

The length of your infusion will vary depending on your medicine and how your body is responding to it. Just to give you a frame of reference, I was usually at the infusion center for about four hours, start to finish. Here's what was included in that time for me:

- Bloodwork. They always did my bloodwork first to make sure all of my numbers were where they needed to be before they started the infusions.
- Steroids and Benadryl.
- Taxotere. My first chemo medication. Often times, Taxotere can cause neuropathy so, to try and avoid

this, I took the advice of my cancer survivor friends and put latex gloves on and then kept my hands in the ice I brought in my cooler while getting the Taxotere infusion. If you'd rather not mess with the ice and cooler, search "ice gloves for chemotherapy" on Amazon; there are lots of options. I never got neuropathy—not sure if that was due to the ice, but I'd recommend it.

- Cytoxan. My second chemo medication.
- Neulasta patch on my arm. Along with cancer cells, chemo also kills your good cells, so you'll need to get an injection to boost your white blood cell count the following day. If the thought of returning the next day feels like too much, ask your doctor if the Neulasta patch (a time-release injection) is an option. The patch is very expensive, so make sure your doctor checks ahead of time to see if your insurance will cover the cost.

AFTER CHEMO EFFECTS

Everyone's bodies respond differently to chemo, so hold expectations loosely. Below I'll share how my body responded, just so you have some frame of reference.

- Day of: Normal
- Day 2: Decent
- Day 3-6: I was laying low because I didn't feel the best. I could still do some things, but I had limited energy and needed to ask for a lot of help. I never felt like I was going to throw up, but I felt a general malaise that kept me from feeling like myself. The closest thing I can compare it to was how I felt during my pregnancies. I was fortunate to feel pretty good during my pregnancies, and only threw up once, but from time to time, I

just felt off. I had envisioned myself hugging the toilet and just being down and out, but it wasn't like that for me. I didn't feel up to being around others much, but I was trying to limit my exposure anyway due to my compromised immune system from chemo.

- Week 2: I felt so much better, but sometimes there would be a day or two when I just didn't feel awesome again.

- Week 3: I felt pretty much normal…just in time for the next infusion. Chemo effects are cumulative and I definitely experienced stronger or longer side effects during my third and fourth cycles. During this time I wasn't bouncing back as quickly, and the fatigue and blah feeling lingered longer.

Some of my other unpleasant, but not-the-end-of-the-world side effects from the chemo were:

- Dry mouth
- Sensitive teeth and gums
- Sores in my mouth and throat
- Rosacea on my cheeks
- Dry skin everywhere
- Dry lips
- Dry cuticles
- Bone pain
- Hot flashes
- Some toenails turning black and blue underneath
- Sensitivity to spicy foods

(In chapter 25 The Beauty Bar, I share products I used or things I did to help with these side effects.)

FOOD RECOMMENDATIONS BETWEEN INFUSIONS

Like me, your appetite may not be the best at times during the weeks in between infusions, but it's important to eat even if it's smaller meals throughout the day. You may find that certain foods sound appealing, while you may have aversions toward others. Listen to your body and be kind to yourself. Even though I was craving spicy food, I had to forego this during chemo because my mouth was extremely sensitive. Remember that even though you will have to give up some foods that make you feel worse than the chemo, it's just a season, and you will be able to eat your favorites again eventually.

As I mentioned before, for breakfast my go-to was oatmeal. It was mild, kind to my mouth and stomach, and healthy. I liked to make mine with blueberries, bananas and a touch of honey and almond butter. I also ate eggs or yogurt with honey and cut up bananas.

Smoothies were my favorite for lunch. I usually put in spinach, almond milk, almond butter, banana, frozen berries, a little honey and ice.

Dinner consisted of a variety of soups, but I had to be careful since my mouth was sensitive to heat as well. Chicken noodle was my favorite, but I also enjoyed ramen, quinoa veggie soup, or just broth. I didn't eat bone broth during chemo, but I know others say it's soothing and full of protein. I also liked cooked veggies, and chicken with brown rice.

Whatever foods were mild without even a hint of spiciness.

For a treat, I enjoyed ice cream, frozen yogurt, and popsicles. Anything cool felt good on my mouth and throat.

THE NEXT STEP

CaringBridge Journal Entry by Tanya Motorin
February 18, 2019

As usual, it's late and it's the night before my treatment. Yes, this is a pattern. It's hard to teach a night owl to go to bed earlier!

I wanted to thank you all for your prayers after my last post. Last week and the week before were pretty tough for me, so it was so wonderful knowing that you were interceding on my behalf. I am starting to feel more like myself again, which I am thankful for. And instead of waking up 3-4x a night, now I'm only waking up 1-3x. This feels like such a blessing. It's hard to be motivated, joyful, and peaceful, when you are simply exhausted. So, thank you for praying. And I didn't ask for you to pray for this, but throughout chemo my mouth and tongue were very sensitive, so I had to do without my favorites like salsa, Indian food, and Siracha...or I would pay the price. Well, last week Nikita and I grabbed a meal at Chipotle and I decided to give the hot salsa (my fave) a try because my tongue was starting to feel better. Well, I'm happy to say, my mouth was NOT on fire and I enjoyed every last bite! This might sound insignificant, but to this 1/2 Mexican, it felt like a really big deal. When it seems like so much has been taken from me in the season, it was great to get something back and to be able to enjoy a comfort food that makes me feel like me.

Well, tomorrow marks the start of the next chapter in this journey. Radiation. I'm told that chemo is worse, but call me crazy, radiation just sounds bad. I was going to start calling it rad, like shortening chemotherapy to chemo, but nothing about this is rad, so I just can't call it that. What is rad is that that I am 2/3 of the way done with Operation No More Cancer. Surgery felt scary and extreme, and left me with scars that remind me of the war I'm in. Chemo wasn't as bad as I thought it would be, but it was still awful, and so hard, and wore me down not just physically, but emotionally. And now radiation. I'm not sure exactly what it will hold for me. Others have told me what to expect, but I'm not sure exactly how it will play out for me.

Even though I feel thankful to be moving forward on this journey, I also feel scared and anxious when I think about all the unknowns and what if's that come with this new chapter. And if I'm gonna keep it real, you need to know that God and I are a little shaky right now. I mean, I know that He's here and I know that He's still in control, but He doesn't feel super safe to me. We've been having a lot of hard conversations recently (well, actually it's been more like me talking about Him behind His back, which is impossible because He's everywhere) and it's hard to be in a tough place with the one that I need the most. Especially now.

Chapter 22
RADIATION

When it was finally time for me to start my radiation, I was relieved, but also scared. I had just gotten the routine down with chemo and now it was time to shift gears and do something new. I was so thankful for my radiation oncologist, Dr. McCloskey, who was absolutely top notch. She went over everything in detail with me, patiently answered my questions, and was just a kind human being extending so much compassion to me. She was exactly the doctor I needed for this part of my journey.

After I went for my initial consultation, the next step was to return for the planning day. Basically they took measurements and created a "pillow" for me to lay on during treatments so that I would be in the same position each time. I also learned how to breathe properly for the treatments. Dr. McCloskey wanted to do the DIBH method which is when you take a breath and hold it in order to pull your lungs away from getting the radiation. If this is a technique your doctor wants you to do, it may take some practice, but you will get it down.

When I returned the next day for my first treatment, I was so scared. I remember waiting in the changing room after I had put my gown on and had a few moments to myself. I couldn't believe that I was about to willingly allow my body to be exposed to radiation. Once again, I was having to walk towards something that I would normally run from in order to be saved. It was counter-intuitive. I was teary on the day of my first treatment, but once I pulled it together (for the time being), the treatment only took a few minutes, and it was already time for me to go get changed. One down, twenty-seven more to go. Before I knew it, I had found a new rhythm with radiation. And you will too.

THE PRACTICAL STUFF

As you go through radiation, your skin is going to become very irritated. There's no way around that. The first two weeks of radiation, when I received my treatments, I had to wear a bolus—a cold heavy piece of rounded metal that covered my breast that was getting the radiation. I thought of it as my shield. The bolus actually "tricks" the radiation machine to think that the bolus is a layer of skin, so instead of going into deeper layers of skin, the radiation only goes to the top layer of skin. Because of that, your skin will get very agitated. Some people blister; I didn't experience that, but my breast had what I called, "Boob acne." I had red dots all over and they itched like crazy. My skin was also very red, hot, raised, even raw. Obviously I wasn't supposed to scratch my skin, so using aloe and Calendula cream really helped to alleviate my skin irritation.

On the third week, they stopped using the bolus, so the radiation would go to deeper levels of tissue. At this point, my skin started clearing up a bit since the radiation wasn't focused on the skin surface. However, by the last two weeks, the cumulative effect of all the treatments began to take its toll and my skin was looking bright red, sores in places, and very angry.

Everyone's skin is different, so obviously your result won't be just like mine, but I'm pretty confident, it won't be pretty.

There's no getting around that. Keep using the aloe and Calendula liberally, and be sure to drink LOTS of water.

With the right care, cream, and gentle touch, your skin will heal remarkably fast. I was amazed that within two weeks of completing my radiation appointments, my skin was nearly back to normal. Based on the way it looked; burned, blistered, and peeling, I thought my skin's recovery would take much longer. It was a reminder of God's incredible design toward healing.

I remember when I was about to start my fourth week of radiation, I had parked several streets away and as I started walking toward 16th Street, tears started filling up my eyes. I could barely see where I was walking. Where was this coming from—after all, I had endured so much, what was two more weeks? On paper it seemed like nothing, but in reality, it felt insurmountable. I just didn't know if I had it in me to keep going. I was spent emotionally, physically, and even spiritually— how could I endure two more weeks? As I walked, I knew that I needed to reach out to someone and God put Nancy on my heart. My first friend. Nancy and I have been through a lot together: lots of laughter and fun memories from family vacations and church camp, but we also were there for each other during breakups, disappointments, and losing our dads. She's like a sister to me. I texted her and told her how I was struggling and needed her help to cross this finish line. What she wrote back brought me to tears (the good kind). We were both soccer players and she reminded me of the grit and endurance that is required of a soccer player. Obviously it's needed for the whole game, but there are some games where you have completely emptied yourself, and yet the ref hasn't blown those three whistles to signify the end of the game. She reminded me to bring this same kind of grit into this part of my journey. I don't have to finish it all right now, I just need to go, "One more minute."

It reminded me of the story from Exodus 17[1] of Joshua and his men who were fighting against the Amalekites. Moses had instructed Joshua to fight the army of Amalek while Moses went up the mountain to hold the staff of God in his hand during the battle. Whenever Moses held his staff in the air, the Israelites were winning. But when he dropped his hands, the Amalekites began to gain advantage. As Moses' arms grew tired and he could no longer hold them up, Aaron and Hur held his hands steady so that the Israelites were able to be victorious. Much like Joshua's battle, I was reminded that this breast cancer battle is not meant to be fought alone. Nancy's words that day lifted my head and spirit to enable me to go one more day.

As you continue down this path of treatment, don't feel like you just need to muster up your strength and push through. Cancer is a formidable opponent and you will need all the help you can get. I feel pretty confident that it wasn't my grit or determination giving me what I needed to lay down on the radiation table once again and raise up my arms. It was Nancy and so many others that God had sent my way to hold my arms up for one treatment at a time. Don't be shy about asking for others to hold your arms up so you can be victorious.

HERE WE GO

CaringBridge Journal Entry by Tanya Motorin
December 9, 2018

Last week my hair started falling out so Nikita and I bonded in a way I never anticipated when we shaved our heads together. We had a good laugh and a good photo sesh, but surprisingly no tears. I rocked a mohawk for about a week and then went fully G.I. Jane a couple days ago—then the tears came. It's amazing how attached we are to our hair. If you think you're not, just wait until you get cancer and go through chemo. No, let's scratch that. I'd never want you to experience this, so just take my word for it. Nikita asked me if there was ever a time I didn't have long hair. I said, "Yes, when I came out of the womb." Oh, and when my mom decided it was a good idea for me to sport the Dorothy Hamill look (if you're too young to know who Dorothy Hamill is, ask Alexa or Siri). I know my hair will grow back, but we've been through so much together and I'm gonna miss it for a while.

PART 5
Hair & Beauty

12/7/18 (text to a friend)

....I'm kinda hitting a wall a bit today. Shaved my head on Monday so I have a Mohawk now, but wear a wig out and about. Even that hair is falling out each day so probably need to shave it all this weekend.

Everything is just sinking in more now and I feel weary and sad. I feel pretty sensitive to what anyone says and I just wanna be normal with normal problems. I wish I didn't have to go through this publicly. I want to just retreat and then return when my hair is back and I feel like I'm not on display while I walk through this storm.

Chapter 23

HAIR 101

If I had to rate the difficult things that come at you during the cancer journey, losing my hair would be one of the hardest. Even the thought of losing my hair made me cry. After getting the results back from my oncologist and after she informed me that my type of cancer responds well to chemo, I was in shock. I was devastated actually. I didn't want to lose my hair, but I knew that I had to do whatever it took to be healthy again.

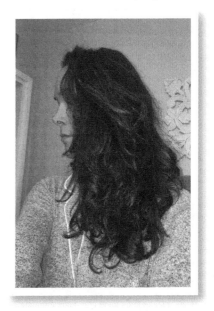

As I drew near to my first chemo infusion, I was getting more and more anxious about losing my hair. I've always had long, wavy, dark chocolate brown hair. Of course I had bad hair days like everyone else, but I usually loved my hair, and I had no desire to let it go. It was part of me. I hope that you won't have to lose your hair, but unfortunately the reality is that a good number of women who have to go through chemo will lose their hair. It's important to know what your options are when or if you get that news.

COLD CAPS

After the reality of losing my hair began sinking in, my mom told me that the daughter of one of her friends from high school had gone through this journey a few years before me. I reached out to her mom to get her number. While I was on the phone with her, she told me that her daughter had used cold caps which kept her from losing her hair during chemo. I felt an infusion of hope surge through my body. I wanted to hear more from her daughter, Debra.

Debra and I ended up talking the next day and then we met up not long after that. I was anxious to hear how effective the cold caps were for her. First, I asked her how the caps worked. They're basically what they sound like, cold caps that are put over your entire skull. They are kept on dry ice to stay frozen and need to be changed out every thirty minutes. Either someone who really loves you can be trained to take care of the caps for you, or you can pay someone from the company to come and do that for you.

Either way, you need to show up two hours before your infusion starts and begin the cold cap process with changing them out every thirty minutes. Then you need to continue this throughout your infusion as well as two hours after your infusion. It makes for a long day for sure. You could potentially be there for a total of eight hours depending on how things work at your infusion location. In talking to Debra and then also doing my own research, I discovered that most women retain approximately sixty percent of their hair.

Debra is a straight shooter and told me honestly that if she had to do it over again, she would choose not to use the caps. This was not what I was expecting to hear. I was hoping to meet with her and basically be convinced that this was what I should do. Now I felt even more confused. She went on to say that yes, keeping her hair was a bonus, but the parts she didn't love were:

- You can't put your hair up in a bun, pony tail or braids
- You can't wear a hat
- You shouldn't wash it often
- When you do wash it, you should use cold water
- You also can't color your hair so you have a sweet line showing your old life and the newer, grayer one growing out
- And when your hair starts to grow back you have the long hair that you didn't lose, and then the short spiky pieces that you lost and are now growing back in

She also showed me pictures of what she looked like before cancer and then pics of what her hair looked like during chemo. In her words, "I looked sick. I couldn't color my hair so it was grayer than usual, and it was thinning. I looked at my friend who had gone through the same journey, but had decided to lose the hair and wear a wig, and she looked amazing. If I had to do it over again, I'd shave my head and get a kick-ass wig."

I wished that our conversation would have soothed all my fears and convinced me to do the cold caps, because I desperately wanted to keep my hair. Instead, I felt even more conflicted.

The thing that pushed me over the edge with the cold caps, was the fact that some doctors are concerned that because the caps are basically freezing the hair follicle and keeping the chemo from reaching this area, that means that the chemo is not able to do its job on your scalp. My oncologist assured me that the possibility of having a reoccurrence of cancer on your scalp is very slight, but I still felt unsettled. Why would I go through all of the madness of enduring a nine and a half hour surgery, four cycles of chemo, and six weeks of radiation, but not let my scalp get the complete treatment. For me, I didn't feel comfortable with stopping just short of the finish line. I needed to know that I had done everything I could possibly do to make sure that I would be around for my kids' soccer games, school performances, family vacations, graduations, break ups, weddings, my Golden wedding anniversary, and spoiling our grandchildren. In the end I chose not to use the cold caps, and that was the best decision for me.

LOSING YOUR HAIR

One moment I felt good about my decision to not use the cold caps, but then the next moment I would start freaking out. My hair was such a big part of my appearance and the thought of losing it felt devastating. My hair was a way that I expressed myself, showed my personality, and my hair made me feel beautiful. Whether I did a thin braid and swept it back, put it in a messy bun, or straightened it for a hot date with Nikita, my hair was like the topper on a wedding cake. The finishing touch of beauty that completed my look for the day.

My doctor said that my hair would start to fall out 2-3 weeks after my first infusion. Exactly fourteen days after my infusion I was sitting on the couch when I ran my fingers through my hair, and a clump of hair was left in my hand. I stared at it in disbelief. This was really happening. Not only was I scared to lose my hair, but I also hadn't picked out a wig yet, so I was afraid I would go to sleep that night and then wake up without any hair. It sounds ridiculous now, but how was I to know how quickly it would fall out? I didn't sleep very well that night, but thankfully when I woke up the next morning, my hair was still there. There were just a few strands on my pillow case. I mean, it wasn't like hair was just falling out and I was leaving a trail of hair everywhere I went, but I knew it would all be gone sooner rather than later. That night, Nikita and I had a family meeting with the kids and I told them that I was starting to lose my hair. They looked concerned, but also took it in stride. I decided to do something fun for them to change up their look since I was going to (unwillingly) be changing mine. I wanted to try and make this time a little less scary for them, so I bought the girls some fun colorful extensions that they could use in their hair and some stick on mustaches for Zion. They put them on right away and we had a good laugh.

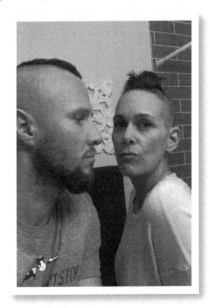

That week, I was careful not to touch my hair too much and I even stopped washing it because I was afraid it would just all go down the drain. About five days later, I knew I had to do something because I was starting to get dreads from not washing it and I felt disgusting. In a way this was a good thing that it pushed me to do the next hard thing. I definitely was scared but I knew that until I started taking these scary steps, I couldn't move forward and eventually through this horrible place.

That Monday, I told Nikita I was ready and we decided to do it together. He shaved his head first—buzzed on the sides with a mohawk. We took a couple pictures and then I let him start shaving mine. As I watched the clumps of hair fall into the sink, I was surprised at how freeing it felt. I couldn't believe that I wasn't an emotional basket case, but honestly I think I was in shock. It felt good to just get on with it like ripping off a band-aid. I told Nikita that I wanted a mohawk and when I looked at myself in the mirror I thought I was a pretty good-looking badass. But it wasn't as fun a week or so later when the hair continued falling out even after we had cut it short and shaved the sides. At that point, I asked Nikita to shave it all because some of the hair had already fallen out and some was just shaved. I looked a bit like a harbor seal, you know the ones with the fuzzy fur in some spots, and bald patches in others? That was me.

NOT ALL WIGS ARE CREATED EQUAL

If you choose the route of wearing a wig, beware that not all wigs are created equal. I had to learn this the hard way. My first trip to find a wig was with my mom, which one of the books I read cautioned that this might not be the best decision, but she was staying with us and helping out during my first chemo cycle, so it seemed better than going on my own. It took so much courage to even ask her if she wanted to go with me. Not because I didn't want her support, but to speak those words meant that this was really happening. I was really going to lose my hair. I told her if she came, there was only one condition, she wasn't allowed to cry. If you knew my mom, you'd know that this was a big ask, but she agreed.

I tried on several wigs, we laughed a lot, because some were just ridiculous. Some wigs I tried made me look like Elvira or Cher, or my mom in the 1950s. We were having a good laugh, but then out of no where, I checked back in with reality and realized that I was sitting in a chair having someone put wigs on my head. *What the heck?* Tears started welling up and I couldn't keep them from spilling out. I looked up at my mom and she was crying too. "Mom, I told you, you weren't allowed to cry." Then we both started laughing as tears rolled down our cheeks. My mom ended up buying me a wig that day that I used a lot, but it wasn't my favorite wig for various reasons. Here are some tips I learned from my wig buying experience:

1. **Give yourself plenty of time.** When my mom and I went to buy my first wig that day, we were in a bit of a time crunch because I had to get back to pick up my kids from school. I felt pressured to make a decision because I was going to lose my hair soon, but because of the time constraints, I started sweating and feeling anxious about making the right decision. I think if I had had more time that day, I would have explored more options and taken time to ask more questions to make sure I was buying the right wig for me.

2. **Don't buy your wig before you lose your hair (or shave your head).** I know that you want one before you lose your hair (so did I), but because I tried my wig

on when I still had hair, once I lost my hair, it was way too big. There are clips or velcro straps to tighten them, but on this particular wig, even on the smallest setting, it was just too big. Ugh. As a result, I always felt self-conscious about it pulling back or coming off.

3. **Find a wig that is not hot or itchy.** If you try on wigs while you still have hair, you won't know if the wig is crazy itchy and hot (like my first one). I was so happy with mine while I had hair underneath keeping it from itching me, but once I lost my hair, it was awful. There was even some rough netting at the bottom that chaffed my skin every time I turned my head. It was so painful and it actually rubbed my skin raw along the back of my neck. It was horrible.

4. **Choose a hairline that looks natural with your skin tone.** I learned the hard way that each wig has different types of netting by your hair line. My first wig happened to have a darker colored netting, but again I didn't realize that until after I lost my hair because when I had my dark hair, it just blended in. Once I lost my hair, it looked so obvious that I was wearing a wig because you could see the dark netting by my hairline instead of a lighter one that would have blended in with the color of my scalp.

5. **PREMIUM Human hair wigs are the BEST.** Even though the first wig I bought was made from human hair, it wasn't a Premium Human Hair Wig (PHHW), so it was made differently. Once I got fed up with that wig, I came back to The Wig Shop, and was introduced

to PHHW. The first time I had one on my head, I was in love. It was so comfortable, secure and natural looking. It was night and day from any of the other wigs I had tried on. PHHW are also made in such a way that they allow your head to breathe, the netting is softer and finer in a flesh color which makes it almost impossibly to tell that you're wearing a wig. The wigs do cost a chunk of change. I bought one for around $700 and another one around $1,100, which is a lot for our budget, but it was worth every cent. I initially thought our insurance would cover part of the cost, but they didn't. Be sure to check on this beforehand if cost is an issue. The Wig Shop, where I bought my PHHW, offers a ten percent discount for women going through chemo, which was such a blessing. If you're feeling hesitant about taking the plunge, just think of all the money you'd normally spend in a year on haircuts, color, balayage, blowouts, etc. You might even save money by wearing this wig (depending on how much cash you normally drop at the salon) and you'll look amazing! You're still wearing a wig, but it'll be a very convincing one.

One last piece of advice... I would highly recommend getting 1-2 additional wigs. I had four total. Each one served a different purpose, and made me feel as normal as I could feel during this difficult season.

WIG #1 *"You get what you pay for"* I forgot to mention this wig because I didn't end up wearing it much. When talking to one of the nurses in the oncology department, she told me that there were some free wigs that were donated by the American Cancer Society for women going through cancer treatment. I went with my husband to try some on (still had my hair) and there weren't really any that I loved.

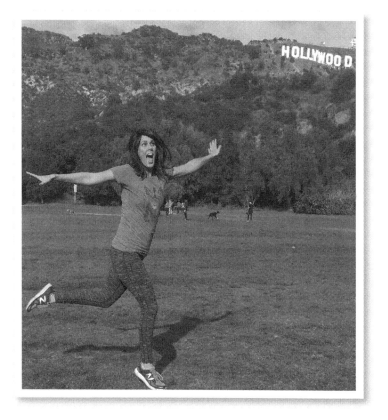

The selection was pretty limited and they were all synthetic and a little stinky—just being honest.

Even though I didn't love it, I ended up getting one, because it was free and I wanted an extra one for a workout wig. It served it's purpose for a bit and I mostly wore it with a hat because it looked so bad. It was nice to have a wig specifically for working out, so I wasn't getting a nice one sweaty and smelly every day.

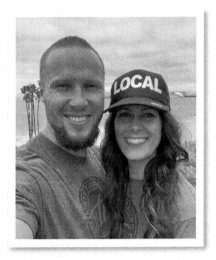

Wig #2 *"Scratchy and Itchy"* This is the one that my mom bought me, so you already know about this one. I wore it for a while as my main everyday wig, but when the scratchy/itchiness became unbearable, I went back to The Wig Shop for wigs #3 and #4. However, this was not money down the drain.

One day I realized that when I wore it with a hat, it kept it in place and made it less itchy. That was great news. It became my go-to for a casual wig to throw on with a hat before I went to pick up the kids from school or run to the grocery store. I also used it as a workout wig once I was fed up with the synthetic one.

Wig #3 *"Tanya"* This was the first PHHW that I bought and the one that looked most like my hair before chemo. With all of the change and upheaval I had experienced during such a tumultuous time in my life, I just wanted to look as close to myself as possible. I wore this wig the most and loved it. People had no clue that I was wearing a wig (even people who knew me well). I loved this wig because it wasn't itchy or hot (I mean it was still a wig so it's hotter than your own hair), but it was so breathable, secure, and comfortable. I highly recommend the investment. The only downside to a wig like this is that it looked so good, I often felt too fancy or done up. Before

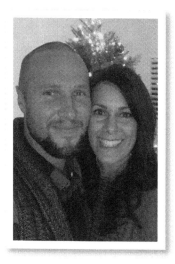

I lost my hair, I would often throw it up in a messy bun or ponytail, which was perfect for my active lifestyle. If I ever go into the wig business, I'd like to create a messy bun wig, because that's real life. Very rarely would a mom show up to pick up her kids with her hair looking perfect (unless you're one of the *Real Housewives*).

Wig #4 "Red Carpet Blonde" When I went to the Wig Shop to buy "Tanya," I knew exactly what I wanted and planned to buy it and leave. However, when Albeir, who was helping me, was pulling "Tanya" down from the wall, I spotted the most adorable blonde wig on the wall next to Tanya.

People had said to me earlier in this journey that I should go blonde or do something crazy for my wig, but I quipped back, "This half Mexican isn't going blonde." However, on this particular day, I couldn't stop looking at this fun blonde wig on the wall. I quietly asked Albeir if I could try that one on as well. When he put it on me, I loved the shorter casual look, but the color didn't seem to go well with my skin tone. As I was sharing my thoughts with Albeir, I asked if he had the same wig in a lighter shade of blonde. He perked up a bit, gave me a smile and said, "I'll be right back." He came back with what he called the "Red Carpet Blonde" wig. He put it on me and I was obsessed. I could not stop looking at myself in the mirror and smiling. I felt like me, but different. At a time in

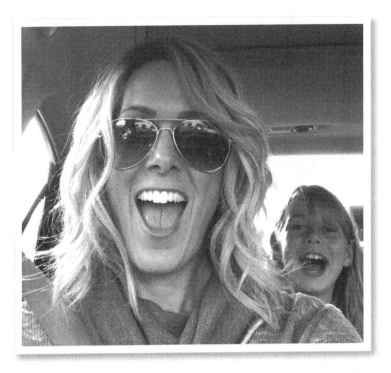

my life when everything felt heavy and hard, when I had this wig on, I felt happy and lighter. It changed my perspective. I told Albeir I was mad at him though, because I had come in expecting to buy one wig, and now I was leaving with two. His reply, "You're worth it."

When I was getting my radiation done, I started with this wig and went for a few days, and then when I came back the following Monday, I showed up with "Tanya" on and the radiation therapists did a total double take. They had no clue that my blonde hair was actually a wig (proof that the premium human hair wigs really are the best). They started touching my hair and looking at the hair line trying to see if they could tell. Anyway, after that when I would show up to radiation on a given day, they never knew what look they were getting that day. PJ, one of my therapists, started calling me "Renee" (my middle name) when I wore the blonde wig. He and Kelly, another one of my therapists, joked that Tanya and Renee were like sisters that looked a lot a like, but were so different. My nephew also told me that I look like Rachel McAdams with my blonde wig on. I'll take that. Hey, if you have to lose your hair, I think it's good to have a bit of fun and maybe get mistaken for a movie star.

At times I felt like a fake when I would meet people for the first time and they had no idea that I was wearing a wig. I mean, I guess that's the whole point, but I usually try to be real and authentic with people. The worst was when I was meeting some UCLA athletes for the first time at one of our work events. The week after we first met, they came back to one of our events. I was so glad I remembered their names, so I walked over to greet them. They were happy to see me, but something felt off. About halfway through the conversation, I realized when I met them the week before, I had on my brunette long hair wig. When I was meeting them for the second time, I was wearing my blonde wig.

Technically, yes, I could have changed to a shorter blonde hair style, but then they would have been really confused the following week when I was back to long dark hair again. That night I ended telling them about all that I was going through. They were so sweet and understanding, and even though it was awkward to have that conversation with people I hardly knew, I felt that I had some kind of control in the situation. I got to decide with whom and when I would tell my story, versus walking through a restaurant without hair, where people would immediately think that they knew exactly what I was going through. The reality was they actually had no clue. Yes, maybe they would know why my hair had fallen out, but they didn't know my story. For this control freak, wearing my wigs gave me the freedom and confidence I really needed at that time. With so much out of my control, wearing a wig almost became like a shield to protect me from unnecessary awkward stares or looks of pity. It was my choice when or if I felt comfortable taking my "shield" down.

WIG CARE

BRUSHING

Definitely invest in a loop wig brush instead of using a regular brush. I got mine on Amazon, but it's The Wig Shop brand. This type of brush prevents poking holes in the netting of the wig.

When you take the wig off at the end of the day, brush all of the hair, but especially the hair at the base of the wig (what sits at the nape of your neck). This area especially gets tangled and matted throughout the day so it needs to be brushed daily. If it's difficult to brush through, it's helpful to use the 909 brand leave-in conditioner/detangler. I bought mine on Amazon.

WASHING

Just like regular hair, human hair wigs need to be washed in order to look good, feel good, and smell good. I know that sounds like a given, but I really hadn't thought about the fact that I'd need to wash my wigs. Albeir recommended washing my wigs every week and a half to two weeks. I would try to stretch this out as long as I could because it was just one more thing to do. However, whenever I washed my wig, it always smelled so good after washing it and it had a beautiful sheen. I always wished that I had done it sooner. Here's how to wash:

1. Fill sink with cold water and sulfate-free human hair wig shampoo. I used 909 brand shampoo from The Wig Shop. You can also order it online. Make the water sudsy and fill the sink with just enough water to cover the wig.

2. Turn your wig inside out and soak it in the sudsy water for 30 minutes.

3. If there is excess makeup on the netting, rub it gently with a soft kitchen sponge or wash cloth.

4. After 30 minutes, turn the wig right side out and rinse with cold water.

5. Squeeze out excess water. Rub human hair wig conditioner in your hands and run through the hair starting at the base through to the ends.

6. Turn the wig inside out and into a ball with hair inside.

7. Let it sit for 1-2 hrs (or longer). I would wash mine after I put the kids down and then let it sit with the conditioner on it while my husband and I caught up or watched something on TV.

8. After 1-2 hours, turn wig right side out and rise out with cold water. Squeeze out excess water.

9. Let wig air dry overnight. A wig stand is ideal, but I didn't want to invest in one, so I hung the wig on a tall bottle of shampoo which did the trick.

STYLING

If you want to blow dry your wig, it would be easier to do if you have a wig stand. I chose not to blow dry mine because my wigs had a nice wave to them after scrunching them a bit and then letting them air dry. Once it was dry, I did like to use my fat barrel curling iron to give it a beachy wave look. If you decide to straighten or curl your wig, you can use hot tools up to 450 degrees.

I also liked sweeping my bangs over to one side with a bobby pin or pulling a section back from each side and pinning with bobby pins in the back. These are styles that I would often do before losing my hair, so doing this helped me feel most like myself. Just be careful with the bobby pins, not to poke them through the netting of the wig.

If washing and styling your wig on your own just sounds like too much hassle, another alternative is to bring the wig back to The Wig Shop or wherever you got yours to have them wash and style it for you. At The Wig Shop, depending on the length of the wig, it costs around $40-60. This is a great option and whenever I had my wigs washed and styled, they turned out beautifully. However, the big down side is that you need to leave your wig there, and it typically took at least a week to be done. Big bummer if you only have one wig and don't want to rock the bandana for a week in between. This is another reason why it is nice to have at least two different wigs.

SCARF, BEANIE or BALD

If you choose not to use the cold caps or invest in a wig, many women decide to either wear a scarf or a beanie, or to go without any head covering. I wore beanies around the house. I found some on Amazon that were soft and cool on my skin. Since your skin is extra sensitive at this time, be sure to choose natural fabrics, like cotton.

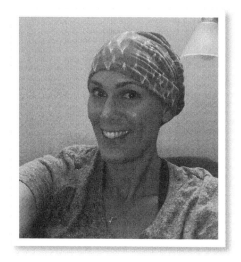

There is no right way to walk this journey. If you decide to go without a wig, let me say that I applaud you and think you are one of the bravest women I know. There is something so vulnerable about losing your hair, as well as your eyebrows and eyelashes on top of that. It was traumatic for me, so it was just too much for me to walk around without my hair for the world to see. Once my hair started growing in, I would go without my wigs at home, but until then, I wore a lightweight beanie around the house. I kept saying I didn't want to freak the kids out, but to be honest, it was also me who didn't feel comfortable. Anyway, if you decide to wear a scarf or go without, I am proud of you and the courageous way you are fighting this battle.

Remember that no matter what you decide to do with your hair, there is complete freedom to do what is best for you. Cold caps, wigs, bald, or beanie... none of these are amazing choices, but it's still a choice.

Whatever you choose, own it and rock it.

Chapter 24

HAIR AFTER TREATMENT

PEACH FUZZ

I can't remember exactly when it happened, but about a couple months after chemo ended, I started to notice some very soft, light peach fuzz growing back on my head. I stood staring at my head in the mirror and touching this new baby-soft hair growing in. I was so relieved that I actually had my own hair growing on the top of my head. Even though it was less than what many babies are born with, it was mine and it was a sign that hope was coming.

Around this time, I popped in to buy something at The Wig Shop and ran into Albeir. He asked me if my hair had started to grow back yet. I took my wig off to show him my progress. I was like a kid proud of her seedling that was finally growing from her Kindergarten science experiment. I was waiting to hear some encouraging words, but instead, he shared something disappointing and unexpected. He suggested that when my hair grew out to about a half inch to one inch, I should shave it and then do that again two more times.

This was not what I was expecting to hear. I asked him why and he told me that when the hair starts to grow back it is damaged, soft, and fine from the chemo. If you let this hair grow out, it will break off more easily once it gets longer. He went on to explain that by shaving the hair three times, it allows time for the hair to come in stronger and thicker. (Side note: Nikita, who grew up in Kazakhstan, always wanted to do this with our kids when they were babies, as this was a Kazakh custom, but I was too sentimental about their baby hair and wouldn't let him do it.) Now Albeir was saying the same thing. I had to decide what I was going to do. Everything in me wanted to pretend I hadn't heard what he just said and to continue to grow my hair out. After all, it had been about four months since I had seen my own hair on my head. The last thing I wanted to do was to shave it off again. However, I also didn't want to keep hearing Albeir's voice in the back of my head as I began to see my fine hair growing in. In the end, I decided to follow his advice and shave it each time it grew out to 1/2 inch. I ended up shaving it three times. It was torture (and set me back about three to four months in my hair growth), but for me it was the right decision. I wanted to do all that I could to have the best locks ever. Obviously I don't have anything to compare it to, and my hair is still finer than it was before I lost it, but it is very full and healthy.

CHEMO CURLS

Maybe you've heard that when your hair grows back it can be a different color or texture than it was originally. This was true for me. I had dark chocolate brown hair before chemo, and when it was growing in the dark parts were more of a dark charcoal color. Not the color I would have chosen, but I had hair so I wasn't complaining. Over time, the charcoal color softened and my hair now looks more like the chocolate color it was before I lost it.

The thing that I was also bracing for was "chemo curls." Once my hair grew to an inch and a half or so, I started to notice some significant curl. My hair was wavy before all this madness, but now it looked like I had a tight perm all over my head. I was hoping maybe as it got longer the weight of it might relax the curls. Instead, the longer it got, the more the curls came out. I'm talking about crazy, Shirley Temple-style ringlets. It was nuts. I kinda have a love-hate relationship with these curls. On one hand, I was thankful that there was some body and character to my hair as I grew it out, however, the curls just wouldn't stop, and at different points while I was growing it out, it was just terrible. I wish I could sugarcoat it for you, but I don't want to set you up for disappointment. There were stages when I looked like I had a permed mullet (it was growing in faster in the back) or other times when I looked like Bozo the Clown as it would poof out on the sides. It was rough. Now if I had chosen to go to the salon to get some kind of "normal" hair cut as it grew out, I'm sure it would have looked much better, but I wanted long hair again so badly, so I had decided to go cold turkey and keep growing it no matter how painful it was. I look back at pictures from this time and realize that some of those stages weren't as awful as I felt. But never having had short hair, I just didn't feel like myself and wanted to get past that stage as quickly as possible.

What kept me going through it all was the fact that I had hair! And it was growing! So, no matter how awful it feels at times, remember that your hair won't always look like this. Your hair may be growing back slower than it did before (thanks to Aromatase Inhibitors, even slower), but it's growing. And suddenly, one day you will look in the mirror and start to feel a little bit more like yourself. I promise.

Once my hair reached my shoulders, the curls began to relax a bit. My hair is still curlier that it used to be though, so it's been an adjustment as I've had to figure out how to take care of my new curls. If you Google the "Curly Girl Method" this will give you some tracks to run on. My friend Mandy, who has naturally curly hair, has helped me with mine. Here are some of her suggestions:

1. **Only wash your hair once or twice a week.** Curly hair is dryer than straight hair, so it's important to not over wash it.

2. **Use shampoo, conditioner, and gel specifically designed for curly hair.** Mandy uses *DevaCurl* products, like *DevaCurl No-Poo Cleanser, DevaCurl One Conditioner* and *DevaCurl Ultra Defining Gel Strong Hold No Crunch Styler.*

3. **Never brush your hair.** Instead, on wash day, get your hair wet and then use a conditioner (doesn't have to be DevaCurl, just one without parabens, sulfates, or silicone) and gently run your fingers through your hair to break up any tangles. Rinse. Then use the DevaCurl shampoo and conditioner listed above.

4. **Once you're done showering, wring out excess water.** Once I'm out of the shower, I wrap my hair in an old t-shirt instead of a towel to absorb some water without pulling or breaking my hair.

5. **Next, I flip my head down and let my hair hang down.** While my hair is hanging, I rub a bit of the gel in my hands and use "prayer hands" method. Basically, I section my hair into quarters, place a section of the hair in-between my hands. Then, with my hands flat (like I'm praying), I glide and smooth the gel onto my hair down to the tips. Repeat with the rest of your hair. Then I cup

my hand under the ends of my hair and keep scrunching handfuls of hair in my hands up toward my roots. After this, I let my hair air-dry. This method gives my curls volume and the gel defines the curls without making them crunchy. There are several YouTube tutorials on how to do the "prayer hands" method with curly hair.

These products have brought so much health and shine to my curls. I especially love the gel. On the days that I'm not washing my hair, I use a spray bottle to spray water all over the top layer of my hair. Then using "prayer hands," take a section of hair between your flat hands, and smooth the hair downward, just like I do on wash day. This brings any frizzy fly-aways back to their curl "families" and helps stretch out my time between washes.

These products are great, but they are a bit pricey. They have them on Amazon, but I ended up buying mine at CVS. Once I used all the coupons I got from my miles of receipts, I saved about $10. Every little bit helps. If you end up trying a cheaper route, be sure to only use products that are free of parabens, sulfates, and silicone.

TO COLOR OR NOT TO COLOR

When I was struggling with my charcoal black color I wanted to just go to the salon and get it colored, but I had some reasons to wait.

Somewhere along the way I had read that you should wait a while after chemo before coloring your hair because the chemicals are still making their way out, and when dyed, it could turn your hair orange or green.

Since green (or orange) aren't really in my color wheel, I was trying to wait as long as I could to start coloring. In addition to that, I also felt hesitant about using chemicals on my hair again. Nobody knows the cause of my breast cancer, but I don't want to be doing anything to encourage the cancer to come back. That being said, I've felt pretty conflicted as my hair has been growing back in. On one hand I'm thrilled. On the other hand, it's hard to not feel like myself when I see my short skunk-like-permed-mullet hair.

I tried coloring it with henna one time, but it didn't seem to change the dark parts of my hair, and the gray parts turned an ugly brownish orange color. I was so disappointed. After more searching, I came across **Earth Dye**, *a* natural effective hair coloring product I found online. I ordered the dark brown and burgundy to mix together and absolutely LOVED it! It is so close to my natural color and it makes my hair soft and shiny! Since it's not a permanent dye, color doesn't last as long as permanent hair dye, so there's definitely more upkeep, and it has an earthy scent, but it's a great at-home, affordable, clean product.

> *Practical tip:* When I used the Earth Dye, they tell you to first wash your hair twice with a clarifying shampoo to remove any build up before dying your hair. I use ***Not Your Mother's Activated Bamboo Charcoal & Purple Moonstone Shampoo.*** Then after coloring my hair, I rinse well and then use ***DevaCurl One Conditioner.***

Because at-home coloring can be a part-time job, I recently went back online to research professional clean hair coloring products. I found a salon in LA called Eco Color Lab that uses **Original Mineral** products, which is an Australian clean haircare line that makes a hair dye that is free from Ammonia, PPD and Resorcinol. Since I still hadn't gotten a salon hair cut since my hair grew out, I made an appointment to get my hair cut and colored. Even though my wallet took a hit, I have to say, I felt like a queen having a professional take care of my hair care needs. And I felt at peace knowing that the products she was using were not harmful for my body!

Chapter 25

THE BEAUTY BAR

Not long after I was diagnosed, I stumbled across the book *Pretty Sick* by Caitlin M. Kiernan[1], which was a great resource for all things beauty-related while going through cancer. I would definitely recommend reading this one. Not only is it practical and helpful, but it also gives you a good chuckle here and there, which is a necessity when you are in the trenches. In this section I share some of her suggestions that worked for me, as well as other products I discovered that were especially helpful during my treatment and beyond.

SCALP

DURING TREATMENT: My scalp got pretty dry and flaky at times so I used ***ASUTRA Scrub The Day Away*** exfoliating body scrub which has has an amazing citrus scent from essential oils and is free of parabens. This helped to removed the dry flakes, but also moisturize my scalp.

FACE

DURING TREATMENT: ***Innovative Skincare Cancer Regimen*** has some fantastic products that I used during chemo and radiation. My favorites were the Cream Cleanser, Pro-Heal Serum Advance, Hyra- Cool Serum, Poly-Vitamin Serum, and Extreme Protect SPF 30. These products helped with my rosacea, dryness, dry cuticles, and protection from the sun. I can't say enough about these products and how good my skin looked and felt. I got compliments about my skin all the time during and after treatment.

During a cancer skincare seminar I attended, there was an Innovative Skincare representative there teaching me and other women going through breast cancer treatments about the effects cancer treatments can have on your skin. She informed us that during chemo (and up to a year after), your skin's defense system has been compromised and you need to be vigilant about using sunscreen since your skin is more susceptible to skin cancer (ugh) during this time. All that to say, the Extreme Protect sunscreen was a lifesaver. The Innovative Skincare products are very pricey, but effective. You can find these products at isclinical.com. If you are in LA, the Reflections Boutique at UCLA offers a discount on their products for women going through cancer treatment.

AFTER TREATMENT: Because of the high price tag (even with the 40% off at UCLA) on the Innovative Skincare products, I couldn't continue paying that much long-term, so I began looking for comparable products at a lower price. A friend of mine who is also a breast cancer survivor, suggested several products to me, and the one I love most is called *Egyptian Magic*. It's made from bees wax, olive oil, and other ingredients from nature. It works really well! It's a little bit thicker than petroleum jelly and doesn't have fancy packaging or fragrance, but it works wonders. I use it at night on my face and neck after I wash my face with an organic wash. Not to toot my own horn, but people have continued to comment on how good my skin looks, which feels great when I feel like I'm barely making it. You can find Egyptian Magic on Amazon. The last time I ordered it I bought a package deal with an 8-ounce jar, 4-ounce jar, and 2-ounce jar. The smaller jar is great to throw in your travel bag.

As far as a sunscreen, nothing really beats the Innovative Skincare line, but I did discover a tinted **Australian Gold Mineral SPF 50 sunscreen.** This has a slight tint so you don't look like a ghost when you are wearing it. On the days that I don't put on makeup, I use this sunscreen. It not only protects my skin without all the chemicals, but it gives some color which makes me feel a little more presentable when I venture out into the world. I also use the regular Australian Gold Mineral SPF 50 Sunscreen for my body. They both have an amazing scent that doesn't make you feel like you are covered in coconut sunscreen. I found it on Amazon and you get a discount if you subscribe to get it every two months, which is about right for me.

I'm also in love with **BEAUTYCOUNTER** clean beauty products which has, "Set out to transform the beauty industry by creating clean, high- performing skin-care and makeup." Since I started using some of their products, I feel more peaceful about what I'm putting on my face and body knowing that it's not filled with harmful chemicals.

One of my favorites is Dew Skin, which is a tinted, lightweight moisturizer with SPF. It's great to put on quickly before I head out to walk the kids to school. I also love the Countercontrol Clear Pore Cleanser, All Bright C Serum, and the Countertime Antioxidant Soft Cream. Beautycounter offers sales or special promotions at different times throughout the year, so I like to stock up during these times to help with the cost. First-time customers get a 20-percent discount on their website, Beautycounter.com

EYEBROWS

Okay, let's just say, I love my eyebrows and I was so sad when they started dwindling. I was thankful that I didn't lose them completely, but they were very sparse. My secret weapon to combat my balding brows, was **Anastasia Eyebrow powder**. This powder is a game changer. Be sure to use a shade lighter than your brows to make them look natural. In the areas that the hair was missing, I used Anastasia's brow brush to fill in where my eyebrows used to be and then I shaped them completely. Nothing beats your regular brows, but I have used this powder for over twenty years, and it is simply the best.

MOUTH

I experienced pretty bad dry mouth during chemo. Using **Biotene** mouthwash as directed was very helpful. I also sucked on popsicles and Jolly Rancher candy. My teeth and gums were also sensitive, so I used **Closys** toothpaste with fluoride which was great. Chemo can cause sores in your mouth and I had them pretty bad. To help with the sores, I would heat up water, add baking soda and salt, mix and gargle for 30 seconds to 1 minute. Try to do it two or three times a day.

LIPS

I like **Burts Bees** tinted lip balm. Again, it does a great job of moisturizing, but brings great color to your face. That was one of the things that Caitlin mentioned in *Pretty Sick*, was that putting on some beautiful bright lipstick could help even on the darkest days. If you prefer the au natural look, use some Egyptian Magic or **Simple Truth Organic honey chapstick**

(I got mine at Ralph's) on your kisser to keep your lips soft and moisturized.

BODY

Stay hydrated! Drink lots and lots of water. To keep my body moisturized during chemo, I used the **Neutrogena Body Sesame Oil, Eucerin extreme dry formula**, and **Trader Joe's Organic Coconut Oil**. None of these were perfect or enough to combat my dry skin during chemo, but I would rotate these or use a combo. Honestly, I think the BEST remedy for dry skin during chemo is drinking LOTS of water! It's God's natural provision for us.

SCARS

Once the incisions on my breasts and abdomen formed scabs, Dr. DaLio, my plastic surgeon, suggested that I use shea butter or coconut oil twice a day. I ended up using both. I bought **Sky Organics Shea Butter** and **Viva Naturals Organic Extra Virgin Coconut Oil** on Amazon. I would rub the shea butter on first, then the coconut oil. I ended up doing it two or three times a day. It really helped to keep the scar areas extra moisturized for optimal healing. Innovative Skincare also has the Super Serum Advance which I used some and this was effective as well.

RADIATION BURNS

I used **SEVEN MINERALS Organic Pure Aloe** and **Calendula cream** each day <u>after</u> my radiation treatment. I applied this combo to my radiated breast three or four times throughout the day. I put the Calendula on first and then the aloe. Use generous portions of both to keep that area from drying out. I had never heard of Calendula cream before, and now it's a regular staple in our home. We use it for cuts, bug bites, and allergic reactions. It's a great multi-use, natural, first-aid cream.

PART 6
Life After Cancer

Chapter 26

BACK FROM WAR

From the moment I heard the word cancer until my last day of radiation, I felt as though I was at war. I didn't enlist, but apparently I had been drafted. That was quite the pill to swallow, but once I got it down, I put on my camouflage, picked up my weapons, and went off to war. There's a reason why people say they are, "Battling cancer." I've never been a part of the armed forces, so I can only imagine what combat is truly like. But in my lifetime, this was the closest thing to war I had ever experienced.

On March 28, 2019, after I walked out of the radiation oncology building for my last treatment, I was honorably discharged with a certificate, some balloons, my purple heart, and was sent home to be a "regular" civilian. This was the moment I had been waiting for. I was done. Surgery, check. Chemo, check. Radiation, check. I had been pushing myself and working towards this day for months. Some days I thought I'd never make it. Yet, there I was.

Soon after, we gathered together with over seventy friends and family to celebrate the completion of my treatment and the fact that I was cancer-free! It was a night to remember. You'd think my cheeks would be sore from all the smiling I was doing and how relieved I felt to have all the surgery and treatment behind me. I was beyond grateful to have crossed the finish line, but at the same time I wasn't sure how to go back to living instead of just surviving. And now that cancer was part of my story, I had no idea how to enjoy my life and not be consumed by the fear of what could have been or wonder about what might happen in the future. Even though surgery and treatment almost wrecked me, at least I knew I was being proactive and facing cancer head on. I was doing all my doctors told me to do to make sure the cancer never came back. Now that I was done with my "active duty," I wasn't sure how to trust God in the next chapter of this story called my life. It felt scary and unknown all over again.

Since I was home and cancer-free, I felt like I didn't have permission to feel anything but grateful, happy, and overjoyed for the rest of my life. In reality though, behind my forced smile, my fear and anxiety was crippling me. When people would ask me how I was doing, it was difficult to know how to answer them. I felt conflicted. I wanted to reassure them that I was fine, but if I did, I wasn't being truthful. And if I was vulnerable and shared about the darkness I was battling, people didn't seem to know what to do with that. They would often hand me the proverbial Band-Aid in the form of a Bible verse or a story about someone they knew who had "beat" cancer. Either way, I felt even worse after talking to them and my fears began to grow.

It was as if I had just gotten back from war and everyone was so happy to have me back safe and all in one piece (kinda), but they didn't realize the tortures of war I was bringing back with me. It wasn't something that just happened to me, it was now a part of me. How could I just put on a smile and pretend like life back home was better than ever? Even though my tour of duty was now behind me, I continued to have reoccurring flashbacks and nightmares of what I had been through. I had difficulty falling asleep at night. Or, I would wake up in the middle of the night because of a hot flash and I immediately had this pit in my stomach when my consciousness caught up to me. I couldn't escape the memories of what had happened to me. It reminded me of how I felt back in my single days when I had gone through a break up. When I woke up in the morning, there was a split second when everything seemed normal, but right after that, I remembered the break up and how my life seemed like it was over. But instead of remembering a sad break up, now my memories were of getting poked with needles, undergoing numerous scans, countless blood draws, anxious waiting rooms, consultations when it feels like they are speaking a language I've never learned, being cut open, gutted, rearranged, sewn up, waiting what felt like lifetimes for results, tattooed, humiliated, nausea, weight gain, hair loss, itchy wigs, burns and raw wounds from radiation, tubes and ovaries removed, and hot flashes—all of this would come flooding back the moment my feet touched the floor. I'm not sure what was worse: living it the first time, or reliving it day after day.

On top of that, I found myself living in the "what if" world that made these horrible memories even worse. What if they didn't get it all? What if it comes back? What if I never feel like myself again? These were the questions that haunted me.

At one point in the midst of all of this, I met with one of the staff from our church because I was feeling really stuck and unable to move forward from the trauma I had experienced. When we sat down together, she asked me to share my story and all of the things that had happened to me during that year of treatment. I shared the above list with her. She started by empathizing with me and acknowledging how awful it must have been for me. Then she went on to share that when our bodies are injured in any way, we experience trauma. She said that it doesn't matter if my body was cut open by a surgeon or injured by an enemy of war, my body perceives it as trauma. She went on to say that even though all of the pain and incisions and measures I had gone through were done to save my life, my body didn't know that. My body just knew that it was wounded, and when you've experienced trauma, you can't expect that you will just pick up right where you left off. It finally started making sense to me. No wonder I was still struggling. I kept feeling like I should be farther along because I could see that my body was healing physically, but emotionally I was just barely scratching the surface. Sure I was an emotional wreck for a good part of that first year, but I didn't have the luxury of having a complete emotional breakdown. I knew there was still so much that needed to be sifted out, but it would have to wait a bit. I had to keep it together for myself, my husband, and my kids. I didn't have time to be in a heap on the floor. And that was okay. I did what I had to do to survive.

After completing my treatment (and even during treatment), I began to experience some PTSD symptoms. It was as if I was discovering shrapnel months after returning from war. I still experience this to varying degrees. Every time I have to go back to the doctor (especially the oncologist), I start getting agitated and feel off a few days before my appointment and a day or so after. If there's a movie about someone having cancer, or the mom getting sick, I have to turn it off or walk out of the theater. I also don't have the same capacity I used to have for sad things, conflict, a jam-packed life, or even simple annoyances. For a time, I was on an anti-anxiety medicine which helped to take the edge off, but it wasn't my preference to be dependent on this to feel okay. My wise doctor reminded me that if I had broken my ankle I would need a cast and there would be no shame in that. So, why was I feeling shame about needing some medication for my mental health?

Since my emotions needed some containment for a season, the medicine allowed me to take steps towards health without being overwhelmed by my emotions.

Unfortunately, coming home from "war" and adjusting to a new normal can be a long and trying process. It can be slower and more painful than you think you have endurance for. That is to be expected. Be kind to yourself as you walk on this road to healing, and invite others like friends, family, and a good therapist to join you as you face the shrapnel. As long as you stay engaged in this process, you won't be here forever—and it won't always be this hard.

Chapter 27

PURSUING WELLNESS

After finishing chemo and radiation, I felt a sense of relief and peace, but I didn't want to just go back to business as usual. After all that I had been through, I wanted to be intentional about how I could better care for my body and my soul. That meant being more selective about what I was putting on my body, in my body, and what I was allowing to dwell inside me. Not only was I seeing the need to avoid physical toxins, but emotional toxins as well. Things I hadn't given a second thought to before, I was now wondering about and trying to think through how to incorporate healthier habits into my daily life.

HOUSEHOLD PRODUCTS

After my diagnosis, one of the first things Nikita and I decided to do was to replace our non-stick pots and pans with stainless steel. I had looked into it a while back, but now I had the push I needed to invest in a new set. I just didn't feel right about potential chemicals getting into my family's food.

I also made the decision to buy cleaning products, lotions, soaps, detergent, and make-up that are either plant-derived, organic, or clean products. At first it was overwhelming to revamp my old go-to's as well as looking at the price tag that came with some of the items. If this makes you overwhelmed as well, take it one product at a time. You don't need to throw everything out or even replace all that you are using. It's important to make choices that help you feel at peace about taking care of your body even if that may be different than what other breast cancer survivors are doing. Unfortunately there isn't a proven "beat cancer" lifestyle or diet, so you just need to make the best decisions with the knowledge you have and then settle in a place where you can thrive and enjoy life.

WHAT TO EAT

As I've continued down the path to wellness, I've been doing more reading on what our bodies need to thrive and also avoid a cancer reoccurrence. Even though I'm not an expert on this, I want to share what I've learned so far as well as pass on resources that have been helpful.

My Cancer Journey, by Dr. Pam Evans, Polly Noble, and Nicholas Hull-Malham[1], talks about how cancer works and what foods to eat or avoid. After reading this helpful book, the first change I made was cutting back on simple carbs which are highly processed and filled with additives and sugar. It was hard for me, but since my health was at risk, I knew it was something I needed to do.

Forks Over Knives[2] documentary was eye-opening and after Nikita and I finished watching, we turned off the TV and just stared straight ahead. Wow. That night I ordered a few vegan cookbooks online and I decided I was all in vegan. I was just so conflicted about what to do with the kids though. I knew that they would full on revolt if we made them eat all that we were trying to eat, but I also didn't want to cook two different meals, one for Nikita and I and one for the kids. I decided to just jump in and bring them with us.

One day I remember spending what felt like nine hundred hours in the kitchen dicing and chopping every vegetable we had in our house for our dinner. By the time we sat down to eat, not only was I exhausted, I was also feeling a bit anxious as I waited for my family's approval. I took the first bite, looked around the table and knew I was done for. I put my spoon down and announced, "You know what, this curry sucks. Let's just say it. I hate it too." At first the kids didn't know what to do, but then we all burst into laughter. I wasn't saying it because I wanted some false praise from them. I really hated it and I was so happy to have an excuse to not have to eat it. In the end, the vegan lifestyle was too restrictive for me, but I know a lot of people who really love it and have made it work for them and their families.

As I continued learning about what my body needs, I was overwhelmed and confused, but desperately wanting to know what I should do to care for myself and avoid making my body a hospitable host for cancer to grow. It felt like an urgent need and very different than my mentality growing up which was trying to limit calories, avoid fat, and manage weight. But as I've begun doing more and more research, I've learned so much more about the types of foods our body needs for fuel. Just like I wouldn't put low octane fuel into a Mercedes Benz, I began learning that my body will look and feel better when I am choosing "fuel" that it actually needs to function best. *Duh*.

About six months later, I was at Target buying more than was on my list, when I stumbled across *The Wellness Remodel* by Christina Anstead and Cara Clark[3]. You might know Christina from *Flip or Flop* on HGTV and Cara is a nutritionist and personal trainer who has also started her own wellness empire, Cara Clark Nutrition. I ended up picking up a copy and as soon as I started reading, I could hardly put it down. Christina and Cara don't just talk about eating habits, but also exercise, and feeding your soul. This book has been such a blessing to me and it came at just the right time. This approach to wellness has been a good balance for me. I have made adjustments that are nurturing for my body and helping it to function best, while also giving myself permission to treat myself from time to time. It's also helped me to understand why you need certain foods and how they help your body to work best. Now I understand that the more colorful, whole foods I eat from fruit and veggie sources, the more phytochemicals I'm taking in, which help my body fight disease. Cara talks a lot about the importance of balancing your blood sugar level by the food choices we make. In addition to this, the importance of moving my body and caring for my soul have been key in nursing myself back to holistic health.

Some of my favorite recipes from the *The Wellness Remodel* are the smoothies, the oatmeal blueberry bars, the kitchen sink salad, and the sweet potato pecan pancakes, but honestly my family and I have loved all the recipes in the book. It has felt so empowering to learn how to eat food that is good for my body and also delicious. When I'm following Cara's food model (with some variations based on my body's needs and aversions), I feel great, I have more energy, I don't feel starved or like I'm depriving myself of something, and I have the satisfaction of knowing that I'm taking great care of my body. I would highly recommend this book as well as Cara's other online cookbooks at caraclarknuturition.com.

I also have learned so much from Vani Hari, who has done a ton of research on the harmful ingredients added to so many of our foods, and she emphasizes the importance of eating organic whole foods and avoiding processed dead foods. I'm thankful for the work that she's done to help the public see the misleading labeling and harmful ingredients in processed foods that can lead to countless health problems, including cancer. Her book *Feeding You Lies*[4], is eye-opening, and her recipes in *Food Babe Kitchen*[5] are delicious. My kids are loving her dishes as well, which makes me so happy. It's impossible to avoid all toxins in life, but I want to take what I'm learning and make the wisest choices I can when it comes to what I'm putting in my body and what I'm feeding my family.

My husband and I are also huge fans of Dr. Mark Hyman, who we first saw on PBS. It's so encouraging to hear him confirming the same findings that I have been reading about in *The Wellness Remodel* and Vani Hari's books. Dr. Hyman's book, *The Pegan Diet*[6] helped me to understand what types of foods our bodies need to thrive. I'm also enjoying his cookbook, *Food: What the Heck Should I Cook?*[7] and his podcast, *The Doctor's Farmacy,* both of which provide some helpful tracks to run on as I'm trying to change the food culture in our home.

Following Dr. Hyman, Vani Hari and Cara Clark on Instagram has also been very helpful to get tips, recipes, and encouragement that I'm headed down a healthy path. The following are the foods I am trying to enjoy, limit, and avoid. I am aiming to do a combo of what I've learned from Dr. Mark, Vani, and Cara. Remember to be kind to yourself (not by "rewarding" yourself with a bunch of junk food), but instead, listening to your body and observing how it responds to different foods. It may feel overwhelming to revamp what you are putting in your body, (I know it was for me), but knowing that I am taking steps to avoid chronic disease for myself and my family, helps to motivate me to continue making adjustments over time that lead to health and life.

ENJOY

- Organic everything whenever it's available and affordable
- A variety of organic fruits and veggies (the more colors the better)
- Pasture-raised or free-range organic chicken & turkey, grass-fed beef or wild caught salmon
- Organic complex carbs (fruits, veggies, beans, legumes, whole grains, limited dairy)
- Unsweetened organic almond milk or gluten free oat milk like Califia
- Healthy fats: organic nut butter (I love Nutzo), organic unsalted or reduced sodium nuts and seeds, organic plant derived oils (olive, coconut, avocado), organic avocados, hummus
- Pasture-raised organic eggs

LIMITED AMOUNTS

- Grass-fed organic whole milk and milk products
- Gluten-free organic brown rice or quinoa pasta
- Organic brown rice
- Small amounts of Himalayan pink salt or sea salt
- "Healthy" treats with sugar from natural sources like honey, maple syrup or coconut sugar
- Dark chocolate (Theo is my favorite because it's organic and soy-free)

TRY TO AVOID

- Simple carbs: candy, soda, juice with sugar replacements, any processed and packaged food
- Unfermented soy
- Iodized table salt
- Highly processed oils
- Gluten
- Enriched bleached flour
- Refined sugar

- White rice
- Pasta
- Sweets with added sugar (only for very special occasions, like when my mom makes her famous chocolate birthday cake)
- Alcohol

I know that it's not realistic to follow this plan perfectly, but when I do eat within these guidelines, I have energy, feel satisfied, and I have confidence that I'm doing my best to fuel my body with what it needs to function best. My goal is to follow this plan ninety percent of the time. Why only ninety percent? Well, I think it's important to find a good balance as you eat and enjoy life, and I don't want to be so obsessed with eating well to stay alive that I miss out on living. So, on occasion when our friends are visiting from out of town, we will order pizza or take them to our favorite doughnut or ice cream shop. But these treats are the exception, not the norm. I also want to be realistic, because there will be times when we are celebrating, traveling, or eating out with our family, and the foods I would normally choose just aren't available. That doesn't mean I go crazy eating Twinkies and Hot Tamales, but I do try to make the best choices with the food options in front of me.

SUPPLEMENTS

It can be difficult to get the nutrients we need on a daily basis just from the foods we eat, so supplements are an important part of keeping us healthy. Using my doctor's advice as well as Dr. Mark Hyman, my daily supplements include: *Garden of Life: My Organics* multi-vitamin and Vitamin B Complex, *Naturelo: Bone Strength-Plant-based Calcium, NatureWise Omega 3 Wild Alaskan Fish Oil, NatureWise Vitamin D3,* and *NatureWise Turmeric Curcumin,* and *Doctor's Recipes Women's Probiotics.*

EXERCISE

Probably the last thing you feel like doing right now is exercising. I mean, it's hard enough to be motivated to keep your body moving when life is "normal," but when you are going through chemo and radiation, or you are recovering and your fears are working against you, it is an even bigger hill to climb. However, I always find that once I get out the door, exercise is one thing that strengthens my body and my soul. Breastcancer.org states, "More and more research is showing that exercise can reduce the risk of breast cancer coming back (recurrence) if you've been diagnosed, as well as reducing the risk of developing breast cancer if you've never been diagnosed." How's that for motivation?

Maybe you already have your exercise routines, but if you don't, www.breastcancer.org/tips/exercise offers some great resources for breast cancer survivors. Depending on where you are in the process, be sure to talk to your doctor about what type of exercise plan is safe for you. I would especially recommend clicking on the "Exercise Safely" link on their website so you don't push your body beyond what it's ready for. Below I've included some additional input from breastcancer.org detailing the importance of aerobic exercise, flexibility exercises, and strength and resistance exercises for breast cancer survivors.

AEROBIC EXERCISE

Aerobic exercise uses the large muscles in your body in rhythmic, repetitive motions.

Benefits: Aerobic exercise makes your heart, lungs, blood vessels, and muscles work more efficiently, increasing your stamina and endurance. It also boosts your mood, helps you sleep better, and reduces your stress. It can also reduce your risk of breast cancer coming back (recurrence), as well as reduce the risks of heart disease, diabetes, and osteoporosis.

>>> My tips: All of these benefits are enough to get me out of bed and out the door in the morning. Some of my go-to aerobic exercises are swift walking, using the elliptical machine, bike riding, running (when I feel especially motivated), doing stairs in my neighborhood, or going for a hike with my family. Since getting my ovaries removed and taking an aromatase inhibitor to suppress estrogen production, my bones are more susceptible to thinning and losing density which can lead to breaks, so all of these exercises not only give me the aerobic workout I need, but they also help maintain muscle mass and help to strengthen my bones.

FLEXIBILITY EXERCISES

Flexibility exercises, also called range-of-motion exercises or plain old stretching, keep your muscles elastic and your joints moving freely.

Flexibility exercises should feel like "comfortable tension." You feel only stretching, never pain.

Benefits: Good flexibility can help you do just about any movement more comfortably, from walking to sitting to bending over to pick up something you dropped. Flexibility exercises also help ease stiffness and posture changes that might happen after breast cancer surgery, reconstruction (especially reconstruction that uses tissue from another part of your body), or radiation. Flexibility exercises also can ease stress and make you more relaxed.

>>> My tips: I've never been great about stretching before a run, walk, or a soccer game, and I think I only did yoga once when I was pregnant, but since I became a breast cancer survivor, I've tried to be more intentional about incorporating stretching into my day. I've started stretching before my walks or runs in the neighborhood, I've been doing some online yoga and from time to time, and sometimes Nikita and I put on some soothing music at night and do some stretching before bed. I've definitely seen a difference in my flexibility and I'm also experiencing less stiffness in my joints.

STRENGTH & RESISTANCE EXERCISES

Strength exercises (also called resistance exercises) make your muscles work harder by adding weight or resistance to the movement. Flexibility exercises, such as yoga, can be strength exercises if you do them quickly, increase the number of repetitions, or add weight to the exercise.

Benefits: Strength exercises can help fix muscle imbalance or weakness after breast cancer surgery. They also strengthen bones, improve balance and posture, and boost quality of life by making chores (carrying groceries, vacuuming) and recreation (playing with children or grandchildren or playing sports) easier and more enjoyable.

>>> My tips: When we lived in Seattle I belonged to a gym that was close to our home so I loved running there and getting to use all of their weight machines and dumbbells. Since it's beautiful most days in Los Angeles, I haven't joined a gym, so I've had to think outside of the box with strength and resistance exercises. Thankfully our neighbor, Sean, is a physical therapist so I went to him when I was rehabbing after surgery. He encouraged me to buy some bands and practice the resistance exercises he taught me at home. Even though I'm officially done with rehab, those exercises are still helpful to continue strengthening my arms. I also use dumbbells and a kettlebell when I do lunges, squats and other weight resistant exercises. Sometimes I'll take small dumbbells on my walks or I'll walk to the grocery store with my empty backpack and then walk back with it full. I love it when I can care for myself and my family at the same time.

If exercise isn't really your thing or you are just lacking strength or motivation, give yourself some grace, reread the "benefits" sections on the previous pages, and then decide what a good baby step would be to get you moving. Maybe even giving yourself incentives when you reach different goals will help you stay motivated. Not only does exercise help your physical health, but it also can improve your emotional and spiritual health. Whenever I choose to move my body, I always begin to feel better emotionally. Between the endorphins, enjoying a change of scenery, and just getting a break from my responsibilities at home, exercise is the "superfood" of self-care.

For me personally, some of my best times of exercise have been with others. Whether it's going on a bike ride with my family, walking with a friend, doing my neighbor's online yoga class, doing exercise bands with Nikita in the backyard, or connecting with God by listening to worship music while I'm out for a walk or on a run, having some companionship makes my workout more enjoyable. Asking others to join me reminds me that I'm not alone. During the COVID-19 pandemic, I had to get really creative when it came to community, so my friend Vanessa and I caught up on the phone while we walked "together" in our own neighborhoods. Even when I'm walking on my own, I like to connect with my long distance friends by sending or watching Marco Polo videos.

The Bible talks about how your body is the temple of the Holy Spirit. I hope that this chapter encourages you to take care of your beautiful temple. Whatever way you choose to move your body, enjoy it!

EMOTIONAL TOXINS

Not only are there chemical toxins that we should try to avoid, but on this journey, we also accumulate emotional and spiritual toxins that aren't healthy to hold on to. I mentioned before that one of the key people on my A-Team has been my counselor. Not only is a counselor someone to process things with while you go through diagnosis and treatment, but afterward as well. Processing the emotions that come up after treatment is a key component of your healing and well-being. For me, I felt a LOT of emotions during treatment, but I didn't have the bandwidth to sort through them all or even feel everything. It felt like a full-time job just trying to survive, so many of my emotions were pushed to the back burner. Now that I am done with treatment, I am continuing to sort through all that is coming to the surface with my counselor. It feels exhausting and it's a lot of hard work, but I know that I can't hold all of this inside of me for years to come. I need to be intentional about flushing out the emotional toxins that could be harming me and keeping me from complete healing. Counseling has been helpful, as well as journaling, talking to God, and sharing my struggles with friends who have created a safe space for me.

It doesn't matter how you choose to do it, just do it. Holding on to the grief, sadness, bitterness, disappointment, fear, and pain won't win you any martyr awards, instead it will eat you up inside. I know it's hard work and not what you signed up for, but keep leaning in and allow others to offer guidance and support in the process.

Chapter 28

SEX & INTIMACY

Ugh. I'm saddened that sex is yet another area of your life that has been affected by cancer. I mean we all know that sex is so much more than just the physical act of intercourse. Sex is intimate, emotional, and even spiritual. It's offering your body, your soul, and your spirit to your man and making a connection that is unlike any other. Sex is one of God's most amazing gifts that He gave to a husband and wife. But since walking through cancer, sex at times feels tainted and hard, and something I can barely muster up the bandwidth for.

Even before cancer, there were always a million things whirling around in my head, trying to distract me from connecting with Nikita. The fight we had earlier in the day, the money tree we need in order to buy a home in LA, where I need to shuttle my kids to the next day, the extra pounds I wish I wasn't carrying around…there was never a shortage of obstacles fighting for my attention.

Once cancer came into our marriage bed, meaningful connection with Nikita became exponentially more challenging and complicated.

Instead of my normal to do lists and processing of the day, now I am also carrying my pain, shame, heartache, and grief. It's beyond difficult to give to someone emotionally and physically, when you feel like you are barely making it through the day and there are so many challenges to wade through in order to find each other. I don't always feel that way, but more times than not after working all day, dealing with the emotional drama that comes with three kids, and still sorting through the lasting effects of cancer, at the end of the day when I crawl into bed, I often feel like I have nothing left to give to the most important person in my life.

In addition to feeling physically and emotionally exhausted, at times I am also still dealing with the spiritual battle within me. Of course I know that I was created in God's image, but there's another voice inside my head telling me that I am damaged goods. Instead of being the "fearfully and wonderfully made" version of myself like David writes about in Psalm 139[1], now I see the scars, tattoos in place of my nipples, and numbers I'm not comfortable with on the scale. All of these factors can make it difficult for me to accept myself. Even though Nikita assures me he, "Loves my body," I'm not sure I do anymore.

If that wasn't enough, because of the chemo, Letrozole, Lupron, and removal of my ovaries, my body official thinks that I'm a blue-haired, 90-year-old grandma. Even though my "estrogen blockade" is good for keeping cancer out, the absence of estrogen also keeps out the moisture. My skin is dryer, my wrinkles are more noticeable, and yes, this lack of estrogen also makes for a dry vagina—and a dry vagina makes for very uncomfortable and painful sex. When I told the nurse practitioner at my gynecologist's office about it, she said it was very normal to experience this. When she examined me, she said that it was dry, but went on to say, "I've seen dryer vaginas." I gave a chuckle. I guess I felt a little better knowing that there are drier vaginas out there. Even though I wasn't winning the prize for the driest, it didn't take away the pain I was feeling every time we had sex. At times it has even felt like Nikita had sandpaper or tiny pieces of glass on his penis when we had sex. Doesn't that just make a woman wanna jump in the sack?

On top of the emotional exhaustion, the pain and mourning our former sex life, every time we did manage to connect sexually, it would take approximately 900 years (give or take) for me to finally climax. Now to be fair, before cancer I wasn't going to win any races in this area. When people describe men as microwaves and women as crockpots in the bedroom, I was definitely a crockpot—set on high, but still a crockpot. So, after cancer I wasn't super surprised that it would take me what felt like forever to climax. But as I started coming out of the fog a bit, I realized that 900 years was just ridiculous. When I began looking into things a bit, I discovered that not only was the Lexapro I was taking for my anxiety probably contributing to my weight gain, but the "decreased sex drive or difficulty having an orgasm" on the list of side effects began to explain why Nikita was having to work so hard to please me. *Are you freaking kidding me?* That's just way too much working against me.

But wait, there's more...I recently connected some dots and realized that I am carrying around a lot of shame, too. I dealt with some of that early on in my cancer journey because I felt horrible that my diagnosis was causing such turmoil for the people I loved most, but now the shame was connected to me feeling responsible for the downward spiral of our sex life. In my head I knew that it wasn't something that I did wrong, it was just something that happened to me, but I couldn't get around the fact that, if I hadn't had cancer, all of the things I just described would be non-issues. I didn't even realize I was listening to this lie until the other night when I had a meltdown after Nikita said to me, "I want you." *Ugh,* I thought to myself, *that feels like such a loaded request. Why would he want me when I couldn't give him what he really wanted or needed? Why would he want me when we have to run a marathon every time he wants to please me?* I don't like doing things I'm not good at, so the thought of getting close to him physically just began to trigger a big fear of failure. This was the last thing I wanted for my most important relationship.

It's messy, I know. I wish I could say that I've figured it all out and everything is amazing now. Sex isn't everything, but it's definitely a huge part of any marriage. My best advice is to keep those lines of communication open with your man. What you are carrying around physically, emotionally, and spiritually is too much for you to handle on your own. It's so important to have an ongoing conversation about his needs and your needs. Bringing your doctor and even your therapist into this conversation will also give you the support and expert advice you need for your body's unique needs. Unfortunately this isn't a one and done conversation, because your needs (and his) are constantly shifting and changing due to outside circumstances, where you are on your cancer journey, and the healing that is taking place. For Nikita and I, we've also had to get creative with pleasing each other because it has been difficult to have sex as frequently as we had before cancer since my vagina feels very sensitive after sex (even with all the products I list below). I'm sad this sacred area of my life has also felt the effects of cancer, but just like I have fought to be physically healthy, I will fight to protect this holy space with my husband. I encourage you to do the same because this area is too important to neglect.

I want to recommend a few products that have been really helpful for me. Obviously we all know that parabens and estrogen are big no no's, since they are linked to breast cancer, so be sure to check the label on any product you choose. Sadly, there aren't any products out there that replace the wonderful work of estrogen for your sex life, but since estrogen is not our friend anymore, the products below are ones that I've found to be the next best thing without the devastating effects of estrogen.

WAY BEFORE SEX

- ***Vitamin E Vaginal Suppositories*** These are a game-changer! Use these three times a week at bedtime. They can be annoying because it's one more thing you need to do before bed-time, but they really make the vagina moister. The key is to use them consistently! I like *Femallay Organic Vanilla Melts.*

- ***Kindra Vaginal Moisturizer*** This product should be used on a daily basis to bring moisture to the vagina. This is a newer product for me, but I'm loving it so far.

- ***Coconut oil*** Using some coconut oil inside the vagina 3x week at bedtime helps moisten the vagina.

FOREPLAY

- ***V Magic*** This is a great product to use during foreplay. It was specifically designed for the vulva and surrounding area to help soften and moisten this sensitive skin as you prepare for intercourse. Initially I didn't really see the point of a product like this because I figured you just need lube for inside of the vagina. However, having the outside skin moistened and smooth (not sticky) has been very helpful for Nikita and I. Also, this is a completely organic product which puts me at ease.

DURING SEX

- *Aloe Cadabra* Aside from the cheesy name, this is a really wonderful vaginal moisturizer and lubricant. It helps to replenish the natural moisture that your body would create. Other products I tried would sting or only last a short while inside the vagina. Aloe Cadabra in combination with the V Magic has really helped my vagina to feel as close to "normal" without my body's estrogen. You can either put some in your vagina with your finger and be sure to get it inside the folds of vagina as well to get the best results, or I've also used a vaginal applicator from a different product to inject the Aloe Cadabra inside my vagina. Having sex no longer feels like sandpaper rubbing on the walls of my vagina (thank God!), and I can actually focus on connecting with my husband instead of just enduring the pain. Aloe Cadabra is also made from organic ingredients so not only does it feel magic, it is good for your vagina too.

OTHER PRODUCTS TO CHECK OUT

- *Queen Bee Vaginal Moisturizer* by *BeeFriendly* This is an organic vaginal moisturizer we are currently experimenting with so the final verdict is still out, but so far it has been great. Unlike V Magic, it can be use internally, which has made sex more enjoyable for me.

I would definitely recommend that you give these products a try, but if you find that they aren't what you need, don't give up. This connection with your man is too important not to fight for. So, even though it may feel discouraging right now, keep pursuing one another and keep searching for products that work for you.

Chapter 29
SILVER LININGS

If I could rewrite the last two years, would I keep breast cancer in my story? Nope. I hate cancer and I always will. However, this season has confirmed the fact that most circumstances or seasons in life are not all good or all bad. This run-in with cancer has been my lowest low, but I can't overlook the silver linings that have cast a sliver of light even on the darkest nights. Though I'm not a naturally "glass-half-full" kind of person, I have seen the value of looking for the bright spots and the importance of acknowledging the good that has come from my journey with breast cancer. Here are a handful of silver linings I've discovered on along the way. I hope they are good reminders for you and a little nudge for you to be looking for your own.

LEARNING TO LIVE IN THE MOMENT

It's so easy to say, I'll do this tomorrow or I can't wait until this or that happens. Before you know it, you've wished your life away. I'm learning to enjoy what and/or who is in front of me and not keep putting things off until the kids are older or we have more money.

TO NOT HOLD ON TO BITTERNESS OR RESENTMENT

There are countless things every day that I could be upset about... when my kids don't obey, my husband disappoints me, or things don't go the way I had hoped. I'm not saying that you shouldn't grieve these losses, but I've been learning the importance of grieving and then letting it go. Otherwise, the bitterness and resentment will take me down.

STOP TALKING ABOUT THE BUCKET LIST AND START CHECKING THINGS OFF
Go on the trip you've been talking about. Splurge. Buy the new dress you've been eyeing, learn a new language, write your book.

ENJOYING THE PEOPLE IN YOUR LIFE
Take time to cherish the relationships that God has placed in your life. Instead of talking about getting together, just get together.

TREASURING THE LITTLE AND BIG THINGS
Look for the blessings that each new day brings. That sounds like a line from a Hallmark card, but it's true. Don't allow the disappointments and obstacles in life to define you. The blessings may take more effort to see, but they are there. An unexpected hug in the kitchen, a beautiful sunset, the sweetest things your kids say.

DON'T WASTE YOUR TIME ON THINGS THAT DON'T MATTER
Social media, arguing, having to be right, holding grudges, or checking off your to do list.

EATING ORGANIC
Over the years I've been tempted to go organic, but I felt like we just couldn't afford it. Now ninety percent of what I buy is organic and I feel so good. Yes, we had to switch thin in our budget, but it has become a non-negotiab family and I'm so grateful.

DATES WITH KIDS
Nikita and I have both been more intentional about going on dates with our kids. Not because we are scared of what might be, but because relationships are valuable and if we aren't intentional, everything else will take up that space.

FAMILY FUN DAY
When I was going through my treatment, we decided to create a family fun day each week so we could explore LA as a family and create some fun memories during a difficult time. Some highlights for me were the Santa Monica Pier, The Grove, Christmas fireworks at Manhattan Beach, movies in our backyard, hiking at Point Dume, the Hollywood Sign, and heading to our favorite plant-based frozen yogurt spot.

MOTIVATION TO GET THE LIVING TRUST DONE
I'm not saying this to be morbid, but cancer really did give me the final push to get our living trust done. It doesn't matter how old you are or what kind of health you are in, none of us are promised tomorrow. It's important to have things in order so your husband or your kids are not having to sort through the legal stuff on top of being there for you as you face breast cancer.

SAY THE THINGS YOU ARE THINKING
I don't know about you, but there have been so many times in my life when I thought things, but didn't voice them. Words of affirmation, words of thanks, compliments, etc. Sometimes we think to ourselves how nice the clean house looks, or how much you appreciate your friend's thought-

fulness, but for whatever reason, we don't say what we are thinking. I have to remind myself...If I'd want to hear it, chances are others do, too.

DON'T WASTE TIME ON TOXIC THINGS

I think you know what I mean, news programs that only sling mud, conversations that talk down about others, arguing, being stubborn. Focus on the things and people that breathe life into you.

YOUR TURN

I know that practicing gratitude at a time like this might feel counter-intuitive, but it can also help remind you of the blessings that have come from this season of brokenness. Find a quiet spot and give yourself some time to write, reflect, and thank God for the goodness He has brought out of the ashes. If it's a challenge to find anything worth writing down, that makes sense. Invite God into this space and ask Him to give you eyes to see the rubble through His eyes.

"*Nothing* makes a woman more *Beautiful* than the *Belief* that she is *Beautiful.*"

— SOPHIA LOREN

Chapter 30
KINTSUGI: GOLDEN REPAIR

*A*m *I still beautiful?* That is the question I wrestled with most often during my surgery and treatment. With my bald head, red angry scars, missing eyebrows and lashes, radiation burns, and a slew of other symptoms I was experiencing, I found it difficult to see anything beautiful in me.

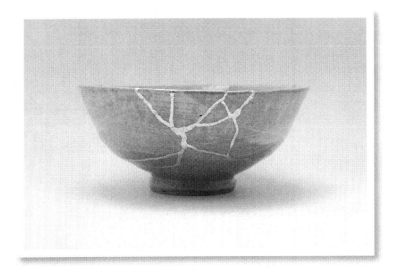

Before cancer, I had my ups and downs with beauty and there were parts of my body I wished I could change, but for the most part I would look in the mirror and see my beauty. I saw my big, brown eyes, my long, wavy, dark chocolate locks that looked good with a beach wave or up in a messy bun. I saw my full, dark eyebrows (even fuller in the 90's) and my long eyelashes that hardly needed mascara. I saw my olive skin tone thanks to my Mexican roots and frequent runs to the beach. I saw thighs and hips that weren't tiny like some of my friends, but I was thankful God made me strong, healthy, and athletic. And when I looked at my breasts, I always wished they were bigger, but I grew to love them because they were "perfect" to please my husband and nourish my three kids. Sure, I had my days when all I saw were my imperfections, but God would continuously and gently remind me to embrace the woman He had made me to be.

I know the woman described above is still me, but when I take a look in the mirror now, I see a different woman there. I still have my beautiful brown eyes, but even they don't look quite the same since my eyebrows and eyelashes didn't grow back quite as full after cancer. And I've had to wait patiently (or not so patiently) for my hair to grow. Who knew how long this process would take? I still have my golden-brown skin, but I often look like a ghost because I'm covered in mineral sunscreen.

One bonus is that my boobs are actually bigger than they used to be (thank you Dr. Da Lio), they feel just like breast tissue, but even the fading scars are still a constant reminder of the trauma that I've been through. And the 3-D tattooed nipples I have now are very realistic, but they aren't the nipples God gave me.

Last but not least, between the trauma, chemo, radiation, removing my ovaries, and my medication, like I mentioned in the last chapter, I've gained more than a few pounds. Even though I'm eating mostly plants and exercising regularly, the scale doesn't budge and clothes that once fit comfortably are now tucked in the back of my drawer waiting for another time (hopefully).

As I write about my current state, I feel teary. At times, I don't even want to look at myself in the mirror. I know I'm still grieving and I'm trying to give myself compassion, like I would a friend, but it's still so hard for me to let go of the beauty I once knew and embrace what God has given me in exchange. How could I possibly be beautiful when I feel so broken, overweight, and old?

At some point in this journey I was stealing a few minutes away from the constant activity in our home to read my latest issue of *The Magnolia Journal*[1]. I read an article entitled, "Kintsugi" that was especially poignant for me as I was in the midst of this struggle to see beauty in the "new me." I learned that Kintsugi is the Japanese art of repairing broken pottery with liquid gold to mend the broken pieces back together. Kintsugi literally means "golden repair" in Japanese, and as I read the piece, I began to gain some much needed perspective on beauty.

Oftentimes when something is broken, I do one of two things: I try to fix it, or I throw it/give it away. I'm always happy when I can fix something and continue using it, but sadly it never looks as good as it once was. This is what struck me about the art of Kintsugi. Not only do the Japanese repair that which was broken, they do it in a way that adds beauty and character that wasn't originally there. Some might even argue that the repaired pottery becomes more beautiful than the original piece. What was once just a broken bowl or plate that could have ended up in the trash, is now a work of art.

As I pondered this art of Kintsugi, I couldn't help but relate it to my breast cancer journey. At first I was stuck in the broken stage. I just kept looking at the pieces lying there on the floor and would weep and weep, wondering how I could ever feel whole again. Not only had my body been shattered and broken, but my soul as well. I felt hopeless. I would often describe myself to others as Humpty Dumpty. I would go to the oncologist, the psychologist, pulmonologist, rheumatologist, the radiation oncologist, the breast surgeon, and plastic surgeon, but "...all the king's horses and all the king's men, couldn't put Humpty together again." I had never thought about how sad that nursery rhyme really was. Poor Humpty would never be the same again. I, too, knew I would never be the same. My doctors and specialists were doing everything they could to "put me back together," but I still felt broken. Yes, I was alive and I was all in one piece (thank God), but the trauma ran so much deeper than I would have ever imagined. Unlike Humpty, I had survived the "fall," but the scars continued to remind me that I would never be the same again.

At the end of the day, I knew I needed God's healing touch. Maybe that sounds cliché, but no matter how good all of my doctors were, deep down I knew God was the only One who could take that which seemed beyond repair and give it meaning and purpose. Why would I think that God would restore the brokenness in the lives of those who came before me, but He would leave me in my Humpty Dumpty mess? Maybe I doubted Him because I didn't think He could make anything better or more beautiful than the me He created in the first place. I wrestled with this and wondered if He would really choose to bring together the broken pieces of my life. Not just make me whole again, but instead, choose to redeem my story and somehow bring beauty from my brokenness—a beauty that would be on display for all to see His redemptive work in my life. I wanted a beauty that when people saw me and heard my story, they would be in awe of the work of the One who redeems brokenness and turns scars into the very thing that makes His creation even more beautiful. I'm now realizing that my brokenness doesn't have to be a reminder of the trauma, but instead, it can be a conduit that leads me to depth and character, wisdom and trust. Not helpless, but hopeful. Not damaged goods, but something more valuable, unique, and sought after. Someone who has a story to tell. Someone who is battle-tested.

I know God is the only One who can redeem tragedy. He is the only One who can come along with the liquid gold to not just repair my life, my body, my soul, but to make me more beautiful and valuable than I was in the beginning. Yes, I think my scars will always make me shutter, and even trigger some of the pain and trauma that I have endured, but they will also be a constant reminder to me of the beautiful work of redemption God has done in me. Like the sun shining through the broken pieces of stained glass, our broken mess can become a breath-taking work of art, not just for us to treasure, but for those around us to be filled with awe and wonder of the God who redeems.

Nothing is wasted with God. Like me, you are not broken beyond repair. I know there aren't adequate words to describe the darkness in this season, and like the back side of the tapestry, it is hard to fathom there could possibly be beauty on the other side. But God sees you. In fact, He's never taken His eyes from you and He is ready to restore your broken pieces with golden repair. If you allow Him, not only will He mend you, but He will redeem your brokenness in such a way that His work in you will be a beauty to behold.

Chapter 31

INSIGHT FOR THOSE BESIDE YOU

This chapter is for your village. The faithful friends and family who are walking beside you as you face this diagnosis. So, go ahead and hand the book to them (or order a copy for them), so they can learn how to love you well during this time.

Hello village...I'm starting to cry as I think of you, because even though you aren't the ones with cancer in your bodies and you didn't have to undergo surgery, chemo, or radiation, you are still feeling it, like a punch in the gut that knocks the wind out of you. I know this is impacting you, too. Your pain and sadness is real. It is heart wrenching to watch someone you love suffering. It's okay, you can to let it out. I know. I wish I could come through these pages, give you a hug, and just sit with you. I know it wouldn't change the pain or take away the diagnosis, but at least you would know I've been there, too. I wasn't always the one with the diagnosis. Like you, I've also been on the outside looking in as my friends or family have been the ones walking through the storm.

With this in mind, this chapter has some suggestions that can help you better care for this amazing woman in your life who is battling cancer. We've all been in situations when we've said or done something we wish we could immediately undo, right? I wish when I was part of the "village" around a hurting loved one, I always said or did just the right thing to care for them. I didn't. Trust me. But to give myself (and you) some slack, it's impossible to know exactly what another person needs at any given time. I know your heart though, it's the same heart I have as I watch someone I love struggling. I know you want to help make things better. You want to make it go away. I don't have a foolproof plan for you, but I'd like to offer some helpful suggestions to avoid some pitfalls in caring well for your friend or family member. Some are no-brainers. Others would be hard for you to know if you've never been handed a breast cancer diagnosis. Consider it my version of "Caring for Your Friends and Family with Breast Cancer for Dummies". Don't take it personally. I'm not calling you a dummy. But unfortunately, there were some people I encountered on my journey that acted a bit like dummies when they said or did inappropriate things. I know this won't make the suffering your person is experiencing go away, but I hope this helps you thoughtfully and intentionally care for her.

WHAT NOT TO DO

DON'T stare at her hairline.
I know it's hard, but please don't stare at her hairline and then try to pretend that you're not. I know that everyone is curious about how realistic wigs look so they want to get a close-up look, but please don't. It's crappy enough to lose your hair, please don't make it worse by making her feel self-conscious.

DON'T keep glancing at her boobs.
I know it's awkward. As humans, we all are curious and interested in the crash on the side of the road, or the breaking news about missing hikers. But, this isn't just the latest news. This is your friend or loved one's reality. Try to have some self-control and not glance down. She's already feeling exposed—like she's

on display, so please don't make it worse. Try thinking about how you'd want others to treat you if they had insider information about one of the most intimate parts of your body.

DON'T tell her stories about your friend who died from breast cancer.
Please don't do this. It completely sucks that you lost your friend to cancer, but she doesn't want to hear about it. She is trying to think about things that are lovely and take captive every negative thought (2 Corinthians 5:17)[1]. The last thing that she needs is a reminder of the very thing she's trying to put behind her. Just because she has or had breast cancer, doesn't mean she wants to talk about it or be reminded of what could happen. There is so much more to her than her cancer journey, so don't go there. Sharing these stories does not make you more relatable.

DON'T give her advice about something you've never been through.
She doesn't need you to tell her how good God is and that He works all things together for the good of those who love Him (Romans 8:28). True? Yes. Does she need to hear it right now from someone who's never been through what she's going through? Probably not. I know you're trying to help, but a spiritual Band-Aid isn't what she needs right now.

DON'T say, "At least...".
As in..."At least they caught it early." "At least it was just in one breast." "At least your hair is growing back." "At least you don't have the cancer gene." These were all comments people

made to me. None of them were helpful. I know you're only trying to help, but your friend doesn't need you to sugarcoat everything or put a positive spin on a really devastating situation. Her world has just been rocked and unfortunately, there are no quick fixes.

DON'T ghost her when she needs you the most.
Don't pull away because you don't know what to say or how to care for her. Because you care about her so much, I know this is hard for you, too, but this is not about you right now. Seriously. If you need to sort through how all of this is affecting you, find a good counselor. Right now, you need to pull it together and be there for your friend. She cannot do this without you. Lean in, even when it makes your heart hurt, and allow God to love her through you.

DON'T send all things pink.
She doesn't need to be reminded of the fact that she's in this "club" everyday. Maybe one day she'll run all the Susan G. Komen races and support every breast cancer awareness event that comes her way, but right now it's probably too soon. Send her something red, or fuchsia, or plum, but please, no pink.

DON'T <u>always</u> talk about it.
Ugh. I would see people when I was out and about, and they were so sweet to check in on how I was doing, but sometimes, I just needed a break from it. Yes, something daunting is going on in her life right now, but it is not her whole life. Let's keep it light. Sometimes she just needs to escape her reality. She wants to hear about your fun vacations, a great movie you saw, or

funny things your kids said. She doesn't want to talk about how her joints are hurting, how much hot flashes suck, and whether or not she'll get approved for the clinical trial. She may just want to pretend that she's normal for a bit.

DON'T <u>never</u> talk about it.
I know, I know. I just told you not to talk about it all the time, and now I'm telling you not to never talk about it. Very confusing, I know. Let me explain. She wants to have a chance to catch her breath and not be reminded of her plight at every turn. However, because this attack is all-encompassing, pretty much everything she does and thinks is affected by this diagnosis, so please don't ignore it. She needs you to read her a bit, and even if it feels uncomfortable for you, to know when to ask how she's really doing and go a little deeper than talking about soccer games, travel, and date nights. Sometimes she might just start sharing on her own because she can't hold it any longer, but sometimes, you might need to draw it out of her so she's not weighed down by the gravity of it all.

DON'T ask personal details about her boobs.
Having a mastectomy or breast reconstruction is so vulnerable, so please don't ask inappropriate questions about her boobs. For instance, "What size are you now?," "Do you still have your nipples?," "Can I see your boobs?" Yes, I really did have people ask me these questions. This is not appropriate small talk for someone who just went through breast surgery. Here's a good rule of thumb: if you wouldn't have asked her that question before breast surgery and reconstruction, no need to ask now.

DON'T ask stupid questions.
"So, did you lose your hair?" Um, she went through chemo, so yes, she lost her hair. I know this kind of goes without saying, but stupid questions are just off limits. She's just trying to survive. She doesn't have the strength to field ridiculous questions on top of feeling nauseous from chemo, dealing with raw skin from radiation, and hot flashes from her "estrogen blockade." Don't know what to say? Just give her a hug. That says a lot.

DON'T expect her to be back to her normal self once treatment is done.
Remember, she just got back from war, so she's not going to feel like herself right away. In fact, she won't ever be the person she was before. War changes you. Trust me, I miss the old me as much as anyone, but I'm trying to learn how to love the new me and she is, too. She needs to know she has lots of love and grace from you with zero pressure to meet your expectations.

DON'T ask what she needs.
This probably sounds like bad advice and maybe even opposite of what you've heard from others, but honestly, when you're in the middle of a storm like this, sometimes it's hard to know what you need on a given day. What she probably needs is for you to stop asking her what she needs. When people would ask me what I needed, it just felt like one more thing that was put on me to figure out. I was already so overwhelmed and, on top of that, I could sense people felt badly that I was going through hell. So, then I felt badly that I couldn't think of a way that they could help me. Does that makes sense? Ridiculous, but true. Basically the best thing you can do is follow through with whatever God is putting on your heart to do. There's not a formula,

so leaning into the God who created her and knows her body, heart, and soul better than anyone, that would be your best bet. If you don't normally talk to God, or you're too pissed at Him because she's going through all of this, that's understandable. The next chapter will give you some tracks to run on.

Now that you've come to the end of this section, you might feel worse than you did before reading it. Maybe you're the one that made the stupid comment or kept looking at her wig, even though you were trying so hard not to. It's okay. I know you love her and she knows that, too. At the end of the day, no one does it perfectly. How could you?

You've never walked this path before and neither has she. Please be sure to extend grace to yourself, but also be quick to apologize for any of the above things you may say or do. She knows your heart and she sees how hard you are trying to love on her, even though you haven't a clue on how to do that well.

WHAT TO DO

Now that you know what not to do, I wanted to share some of the things friends and family did that cared for me deeply. I also added some things I wish others would have done for me. Obviously everyone is different, but if your person is in the middle of this battle, these might be tangible ways to show what you wish you could express with your words. I hope these ideas can help you not feel quite as helpless. Just the fact you are reading this and wanting to know how to care for your person says how much she means to you. She's lucky to have you.

TEXT

Often times God will bring your friend to mind throughout the week or throughout the day. When He does, reach out with a simple text. I know it can feel hard to come up with just the right words to say, but that's not what your friend is expecting. She just wants to know that she's not alone in this and there are people who are thinking of her, love her, and are with her. Example text: "Just wanted you to know that I love you, I'm thinking of you this morning, and I'm with you in this battle." Done. She's cared for.

PRAY

I know it may sound like a Sunday School answer, but prayer is actually good for you and for her. Here's some easy ways/times to pray for her:

- Put your friend on your prayer list
- Set a reminder on your phone to pray for her at a certain time each day
- Ask your friends in your Bible study to pray
- When you wake up in the middle of the night to go pee, see that as an opportunity to pray for her
- When you run into your friend at the grocery store or at school pick up, let her know that you've been praying for her
- Ask if there's anything specific she wants you to be praying for this week
- When you see her in person, ask if you can pray for her then and there

Okay, I hear some of you already saying, but I don't know what to pray for. Start by listening—she will give you some clues about what she's currently battling. Here's a few other specifics to pray for: peace, complete healing, courage, strength, that she would be kind to herself, that the cancer would not return, joy in the midst of such a difficult time, her marriage, her husband, her kids, and anything else God puts on your heart.

CARE FOR HER KIDS

When you are at Target with your kids and they beg you to get something from the dollar section, buy it for them, and then buy a couple extra for your person's kids. They are feeling all the strain, sadness, and fear that their mom and dad are carrying around. Even if they don't express it, this is heavy for them. I know some candy and a $1 light up bouncy ball won't take the cancer away, but it will help those kids to know that someone sees their pain and fear, too. And when your person sees that her kids are being cared for, she feels cared for, too.

SEND A CARE PACKAGE

It can be especially challenging for those who are far from family or friends while going through breast cancer. Sending a care package is a beautiful way to show her that, even though she is out of sight, she is definitely not out of mind. I had friends send blankets, tea, a gift card, chocolate, or just something to make me smile. One of my favorites was a mug that said, "Strong and Beautiful." I still treasure the mug, and I tend to reach for that one on the days when it's hard to believe that.

FLOWERS

I'm not talking about the ones that will break the bank. I'm saying, clean out that pasta jar, take off the label, go in your backyard and clip some of the beautiful garden roses or Bougainvillea you've been admiring from your kitchen window. Drop them off on her front doorstep with a Post-It note saying, "I love you." If you're all the way across the country and can't just stop by, do what my friend Lindsay did and send a beautiful bouquet from farmgirlflowers.com

CALL

There are a million reasons you can come up with to not call her. "She's too exhausted to talk to anyone." "I can't relate to what she's going through, so what would I say?" "If I were going through this, I'd just want to crawl into a hole and come out when everything was back to normal." "It's too hard for me to hear about all that she's going through. It's breaking my heart." There are so many more that I could list, but the reality is, she's your daughter or sister or mom or friend, and she needs you. When you get the courage to finally pick up the phone and call her, here are a few scenarios that could happen:

1. She won't pick up or call you back because she's just trying to survive, but she will be encouraged by your sweet voicemail and reminder that there's no need to call you back.

2. She won't pick up, but she'll call you back later and you'll get a better picture of what she's dealing with and know how to pray for her.

3. She'll pick up and you will have a great convo. She'll feel loved and you'll give her a few minutes to think about something other than the hell she's living.

All that to say, go ahead and call her. And if she doesn't pick up, leave a short message letting her know that you were thinking of her and that there's no pressure to call back.

KEEP CHECKING IN

A lot of people rise to the occasion in the midst of a crisis, but then once someone is "out of the woods," those around her go back to business as usual. The reality is, your girl needs you just as much for the year or two after she finishes treatment as she did when she was in the thick of it. My counselor, who is a breast cancer survivor herself, says to give it at least three years.

GET IN THE PIT

Sometimes we want to love on people from afar where it feels safe, but what she really needs is people who aren't afraid to draw near and enter into her pain. You don't need to fix it, just be with her. I could never express it as well as Brené Brown. Go to YouTube, and search for "Brené Brown on Empathy."[2] So insightful and practical.

JUST DO IT

Instead of asking her what she needs, just think about what you'd want and do that. If you ask, she may feel bad and not want to be a burden to you. So tell her you'd like to:

- Clean her house or send someone from a cleaning service, then ask, "When is good time to do that?"

- Take her kids to the park for the afternoon, then ask, "What day works this week?"
- Bring her dinner on Friday, then ask, "Do you want Italian or Mexican?"

Then do the same thing next week or next month.

GOODIE BASKET

When you are already at Target getting all the items you didn't have on your list, throw some goodie basket items in your cart too. *People* magazine, *Napoleon Dynamite* on DVD, popcorn, a face mask, dark chocolate. She will love the chance to laugh, care for herself, and escape reality for a few hours.

BRING DINNER

While your friend or family member is recovering from surgery or going through treatment, bringing dinner is a practical way to care for her and her family. It could be your family's famous lasagna, or a rotisserie chicken, some garlic bread, and a prepackaged salad from the store. Often times when I am making soup or chili for my family I will just double the recipe so I don't have to go to the trouble of making an extra meal. No need for anything fancy. If you are far away, send an electronic gift card for her favorite restaurant, or pick one up at the grocery store and send it with a hand written note. Even though the obvious time to send a meal is during recovery or treatment, I would also encourage you to bring a meal even weeks or months after she is done with treatment. Just because she's done with formal treatment doesn't mean she has the bandwidth to carry the same load she did before her diagnosis.

Any meal she doesn't need to shop for, prepare, and cook is an easy way to lighten her load during or after treatment.

SEND ICE CREAM

Two of the best surprises during my treatment were when friends living in Rwanda and Seattle sent ice cream. Okay, the ice cream didn't actually come all the way from Rwanda, but my friends I met in Ohio (who have been through their own cancer journey), and are now living in Rwanda, ordered ice cream from Graeter's (the best ice cream in Ohio), and had it sent to me unexpectedly with a note that said, "Ice cream makes everything better." Then Nikita had our friends in Seattle send salted caramel from Molly Moon's Ice Cream for our family. They put it on dry ice, sent it overnight, and the next day we were loving life.

There are so many other things you can do to love on your person. You can do exactly what I wrote, or you can take my ideas and tweak them to cater to the things you know will really care for your person.

MAN TO MAN

I asked Nikita to write a bit to the man in your life who is faithfully standing beside you through this difficult time. Reading his words brings tears to my eyes, and at the same time, so much encouragement. I hope you can pass this on to your hubby, boyfriend, or best bud so he can be encouraged too.

The kids were running around in the backyard and I was in the middle of packing up the last of our things before our move, when my wife texted me from her follow-up mammogram appointment to say that the doctor was pretty certain it was cancer. I stared at the screen and didn't know what to do. I was in complete shock. The words weren't even registering. I had been in task mode getting ready for the movers to come, and now I was having to shift gears and think about a life-threatening disease in my wife's body. I honestly didn't know how to process it. I'm a typical guy who compartmentalizes everything and multitasking is my weakness, so having to hold the stress of the move at the same time that I'm absorbing the news that my wife had cancer was too much for me. There were a million questions that immediately flooded my mind. What does this mean? What kind of cancer does she have? How advanced is it? Should I be freaking out? All of the unknowns felt scary and fear was starting to seep in. I wondered how this was happening and how we would get through it.

Later, my shock turned to anger toward God. How dare He allow this to happen to our family in the midst of us moving from Seattle to LA so that we could serve Him at UCLA. This was not in the plan and I was pissed. I wanted to hit something. I knew that this wouldn't help, but what else could I do? I'm wired to fix things and I desperately wanted to fix this, but I couldn't. I wanted to make it all go away, but my hands were tied. I was at God's mercy. I had to trust, even though I didn't understand, and I wasn't sure that He was trustworthy.

There aren't even words to describe how much I despise cancer and the havoc that it has brought to my family, and now yours. It's not okay. The pain, anger, fear, anxiety, uncertainty, and chaos you are experiencing is legit. I wouldn't wish it upon my worst enemy. I know you don't know me and I don't know you, but can I just say that I hate that you and your family are facing this horrible disease? I get it man.

It's a nightmare I know you wish you could wake up from.

When Tanya asked me to share with you and other husbands with wives battling breast cancer, I wanted to help, but I didn't know where to start or what to say. I mean who am I to share anything? I'm not a doctor or an expert on how to survive or thrive during trauma. I'm just a husband who barely made it through some days, and completely lost it on others. So no, I haven't figured out the right way to navigate all this crap, but, because of the fact that I'm a little bit ahead of you on this journey, I guess that qualifies me to share my two cents. I know that nothing I write has the power to change your circumstances, but I hope that my perspective and insight might help you in some way.

For starters, I want you to hear that even though cancer isn't in your body, you are also battling cancer. This diagnosis isn't just affecting your wife, it is reaching you and your kids. I know this probably sounds like a no-brainer, but I think it's important to acknowledge the fact that you are also fighting your own battle. Normally there are two people running your household and keeping your family afloat...now the majority falls on you. I don't know how your family roles were divided up before, but now for the most part you will become the bread winner, the chef, the chauffeur, the referee, the organizer, the calendar keeper, and the CaringBridge blogger. On top of all that, you also need to be the encourager, and the one to listen and support your wife and kids when this emotional battle is weighing them down. Are you overwhelmed yet?

I'm not sharing all of this to raise your anxiety level, but I do want you to take a step back and recognize what is being asked of you is a lot. It's going to be rough and you're going to want to hit something too when you realize that you can't do the impossible task in front of you. You can't fix it and even though you love your wife and kids more than words can express, you cannot do it all. It's time to call in the troops. It's time to ask for help. I know that a guy asking for help is very similar to a guy asking for directions, but it's time to suck it up and turn to your extended family members, friends, and neighbors for help to carry you all through this time. This is not a one-person battle. Speaking from experience, I know it's hard to ask for help, but you need to. Doing it all on your own is not sustainable. Plus, those around you are feeling helpless and wanting to know practical ways to love on you guys. So, kill two birds with one stone by letting them help and lightening your load.

Once I got some people to help me carry the weight, I had more space to sort through the anger that was making me want to hit something and the despair that was causing some deep depression (even though I didn't realize it yet). It's so important to recognize that what you are feeling and experiencing also matters. Yes, your wife has (or had) cancer. That's a big deal. It's earth-shattering. That kind of trauma doesn't just work itself out over night. As a result, you will obviously have a lot to process and to come to terms with as well. As those waves hit you, it's so important to not let your grief, anger, fear, and heartache get lost in the midst of being there for everyone else. It's also not helpful to sweep it under the rug, because it won't go away on its own. If there's only one thing you can take away from what I'm sharing, this should be it: You have to take care of yourself so that you can take care of her...and them. Like the flight attendant reminds you on every flight—you've got to put your own mask on first. You will have nothing to give them if you aren't caring for yourself, too. No one can read your mind though, so speak up and share what you need as well. You will be better equipped to love and care for your wife and kids in meaningful ways when you are coming from a place of overflow instead of depletion.

So, what does this look like? How do you take care of yourself when your wife and kids need you more than ever? Isn't that selfish?

Absolutely not. Trust me, you will be a better version of yourself by filling up your cup before you have to pour out! Here are some tangible ways that I cared for myself throughout this journey:

- **Surfing.** Escaping to the beach gave me time away from the house and away from cancer. I know that I can't really run away from cancer, but the change of scenery was good for my soul and it allowed me to catch my breath, connect with friends, and connect with God.

- **Working out.** Working out was also a great release for me. Going for a run, doing the stairs or lifting hard gave me space to blast my AirPods while praying and crying out to God. I didn't want to be a mess in front of my wife, so this space was good for me to exhale and express my anger and fear.

- **Stopping for pastries on the way home from surfing.** I have a crazy sweet tooth, and yes, sometimes I run to food to bring me comfort in stressful times (although I'm not promoting that as the best way to cope), but some days, a pastry from my favorite bakery was the bright spot I needed to head back into the darkness.

- **Doing an add-on.** Tanya talked about it in the book, but she coined the term "Add-on" to something I just do instinctively. Often times while I was out picking up her prescriptions or groceries for the family, I would add-on something small for myself. Sometimes I'd stop at Nordstrom Rack to find some deals or get my caffeine fix at Alana's Coffee on my way home from Costco. I wasn't going out and doing something just for me (although that's okay at times, too). Instead, while I was out serving my wife and my family, I made sure to care for myself, even if it was in the smallest way.

- **I found trusted friends I could turn to.** Being new to Los Angeles made it tough at the beginning, but God quickly provided men who came alongside me during this difficult time. I needed space to be weak, vulnerable, and to let my guard down. I needed these friends to be intentional with me, speak life into me, and allow me to process things (if I wanted to), and not have it all figured out. I don't know what I would have done without friends to work out with, grab coffee, enjoy time around our fire pit, and my "Dawn Patrol" friends who I could catch some waves with. Sometimes we would talk about cancer, but most of the time it was just nice to have a break from it. These friends felt like God's lifeline in the midst of the storm.

- **Get some professional help.** I benefitted so much from talking to our counselor. One thing she helped me realize through our conversations was that all of the anger and numbness I was experiencing was coming from a place of helplessness. My wife that I love so much, was going through it and I couldn't do anything. It was killing me. It felt like everything was out of my control. Talking with her didn't change my circumstances, but it gave me some much needed validation, empathy, an outside point of view, and space to be broken and grieve.

That's all I got. I hope that my perspective gives you some encouragement, help, or maybe permission to feel and express the anger and fear you are wrestling with inside. If nothing less, I hope my story reminds you that you're not alone in this.

— Nikita (Tanya's husband)

FROM MY KIDS TO YOURS

If you have kids, I'm sure they are amazing and resilient just like mine, but underneath their sweet and strong exterior, there are lots of thoughts, questions, and fears as they try to absorb the fact that their mom has (or had) cancer. This section is for them; our sweet heroes. Here are some thoughts from my kids that I hope will spark some helpful and healing conversations between you and your kids.

THOUGHTS FROM HOPE (AGE 12)

At different times, we all go through really hard things in life. When I first heard that my mom had breast cancer, I really didn't know what was going to happen. I felt overwhelmed. It was a hard conversation and after she told us, I didn't know what to do, so I gave my mom a big hug. I know she needed it and I did, too.

About a month or so later, my mom had to go to the hospital to have her surgery. My grandma came to stay with us since my dad wanted to be there for my mom most of the time. She was in the hospital for about a week. Our two aunts and my uncle came to stay with us and help also, but it was still a stressful time for me, Sophia, and Zion.

While my mom was still in the hospital, my dad told me that we were going to go there to see her. I was so excited to see my mom because I missed her so much, but I was nervous to know if she would look different or anything. I was relieved when we finally saw her and she looked like my same ol' mom. We brought her an Ice Blended from Coffee Bean (our family is in love with them), It was really good to catch up with her and see her beautiful face, and to be with her again!

A few days later, my mom came home! She was very weak and we had to take care of her but I didn't mind. Since my mom couldn't cook for us at the beginning, it was so great when our school sent out an email to all the families that go there and said that we could use some help with meals. It was so great that every other day all different families would bring meals for our family to enjoy! It was very sweet of them!

My aunt also made some really good meals for us.

A few weeks after my mom was back home, we had another family meeting and my mom shared the saddest news. She told us that since she needed chemo to make sure the cancer didn't come back, she was going to lose her hair! I didn't know why it had to happen, but my mom said once her hair started falling out that she was going to shave all her hair off. When I heard this, I really wanted to start crying, but I didn't. I don't know why. I guess I was in shock.

A few weeks after this, my mom's hair started falling out, so she and my dad decided it was time to cut her hair. The next morning my mom and dad told us that my dad gave her a mohawk! At first she was wearing a beanie around the house because my brother and sister and I said we didn't want to see her shaved head. But, after a day or two, Sophia and Zion changed their minds and decided they wanted to see her hair. I felt hesitant, but then I decided that I wanted to see it, too. We were all so surprised to see our mom with a mohawk! It was so awesome. And even better, our dad decided to do the same hairstyle as our mom. I was so happy, but so sad at the exact same time.

Not long after that, even the hair from my mom's mohawk fell out, so my mom bought some different wigs she could wear. It was so awesome because I am the only one in our family that has blonde hair, and my mom actually bought a wig that was blonde!! Haha. It was fun to have my mom and I look more alike! She eventually ended up with about five wigs and we loved trying them all on. Our dad and brother were so funny when they put the wigs on.

After chemo, my mom also had to go to radiation every day for six weeks. It didn't seem as hard as chemo, but she was still really tired.

Finally, my mom's hair started to grow back. She was so excited and I was too. The very surprising thing was that her hair was so curly. I wasn't expecting that, because her hair was just wavy before, but it's so pretty now that it has a different style. Even though my mom looked different with short hair, she was still my mom and I felt happy for her. Life was starting to feel normal again...my mom could cook, she took care of things, and she started going on her morning walks! About a year later, she stopped wearing her wigs, and now her hair is getting so long. It's not as long as it used to be, but it's getting there.

My mom's journey was pretty hard and I felt like I was the one going through it too just by being her daughter. I know you must feel the same way. I know it's really really hard, but everything will be fine. Life can be so rough, but I've learned that going through the hard times reminds me to love the good parts even more.

God is within her, she will not fall. God will help her at break of day. — Psalm: 46:5[3]

Q & A WITH SOPHIA (age 10) and ZION (age 8)

What kinds of feelings ran through your heart when we had a family meeting and I told you that I had breast cancer?

S: *I was thinking, "What's breast cancer?" After we talked more as a family, I knew that it was something bad that you didn't want to have in your body. I was kind of scared when my mom told us that she had to have surgery to get it out.*

Z: *I was sad because my mom was going to have to be in hospital and I would miss her. I also was scared because I didn't understand what cancer was.*

What was the hardest part for you when I was going through my cancer journey?

S: *It was hard for me when my mom was in the hospital and she couldn't be with me. I was used to always having her at the house so I felt sad when she couldn't put me down at night.*

Z: *It was hard that my mom couldn't play with me like she normally did and I was sad because she couldn't lay down with me at night when she was still healing from her surgery.*

What made that time not as horrible for you?

S: *It was fun when my dad shaved my mom's hair before it started falling out completely and she had a mohawk! We had fun messing around with her hair and taking pictures. Also, when my mom was going through her treatments, we started having "Family Fun Day" on Tuesdays and we would all do something fun together as a family. This was nice because we got to spend more time with my mom and dad* exploring *Los Angeles. One more thing that made it not so horrible was when we had special family members come to take care of us. I loved getting to spend that extra time with my Nana, Aunt Tara, Aunt Irene, and Uncle Todd. I especially loved getting to have the special treats they made or brought for us.*

Z: *I liked going on dates with my mom and special time with her.*

If your friend told you that she just found out that her mom has cancer, what would you tell her?

S: *I would tell her that I think everything will be alright because my mom went through breast cancer, and she is fine now. I would also tell her that it's scary sometimes, but other times it feels okay.*

Z: *I would tell my friend that I hope her mom feels better. I would also say, that this is scary, but it won't always be this scary.*

What advice do you want to give to other kids going through what our family has been through?

S: *Sometimes it's good to talk to a friend about it, you don't have to keep it all to yourself and feel stressed or worried. Sometimes I would talk to my friend Audrey about my mom's different colored wigs and how that wasn't her real hair. I also told her that my dad looked like Jesus when he tried on one of her wigs and we laughed a lot about that.*

Z: *Enjoy every day with your mom and try not to worry about tomorrow.*

What encouragement do you have for kids in your shoes?

S: *It's important to just take one day at time and see how it feels, that's what I did and it helped me. Also, if you need to talk to someone about it, don't be afraid to tell them how you feel. God helped our family by having people bring us meals, pray for us, and support us, so I know that He will take care of you too.*

Z: *It's okay to feel what you're feeling. Sometimes you might feel sad and other times you might feel normal, and that's okay.*

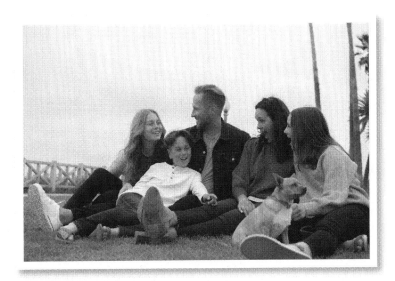

THANK YOU

CaringBridge Journal entry by Tanya Motorin
April 21, 2019

Last Saturday, over seventy people gathered at our house to eat tacos, visit, laugh and cry, but most of all to celebrate the fact that I am cancer free!!! My heart was so full as I looked around at so many of the friends and family that God had used to care for me over the last nine months. It was such a beautiful night that I will always hold dear.

As we gathered, I shared that many times throughout the last nine months, God brought to mind the account of the paralytic in the Bible who was carried to Jesus by his four friends. I've always loved this story, and because of all that I've been through this year, this story resonates with me in an even deeper way. If you are familiar with the story, you'll remember that when the men got to the house where Jesus was teaching, it was so crowded that there was no room for them to get inside. Determined to get their friend to Jesus, the friends made a hole in the roof and lowered their friend through it so that Jesus could heal him. The story goes on to say that when Jesus looked at them (his friends) and saw their bold faith, then he healed the man and he picked up his mat and walked home that day.

Since July, you all have been the ones taking turns carrying a corner of my stretcher as you brought me to Jesus. When I didn't want to talk to God (because I wasn't sure that He was safe and I didn't know if we could be friends), and I didn't feel like reading His word, He found a back door into my heart. That was you. So, not only were you carrying me to Him, He was also using you to reach me. If there was one way that God moved and showed up the most for me throughout this journey, it was through each of you. Even though I wanted to unfriend Him at times, I couldn't deny God's presence and His goodness because it was so evident in the each of you. You have been the ones carrying me to Jesus when I didn't think I could go on and I was paralyzed by fear, pain, grief, trauma, sadness and depression. So, even though I know that my words will never do justice to all the ways that you have loved and served me and my family, I want to try to thank you. So, this is my attempt at one massive thank you note for those of you (you know how you are) who prayed, gave, reached out, and showed up. THANK YOU for...

- Sending care packages filled with coffee, chocolate, and yes even ice cream from Seattle.
- Giving books, blankets, candles, a juicer, did I say chocolate? :-) , and so many other thoughtful gifts that showed that you saw us and loved us.
- Gift cards that gave me a break from having to answer the question, "Mom, what's for dinner?"
- Taking time out of your day to send a card and share your heart with me.
- Praying. Your prayers have sustained me.
- Crying with me.
- Bringing a meal. Or two.

- Taking my kids for a play date.
- A shopping spree at Lululemon.
- Cleaning my house.
- Babysitting my kids so I could have a date with my hubby.
- Being intentional with my husband and kids, because this journey hasn't just been mine. It has affected all of us.
- *Removing my cancer.*
- Handing me a Kleenex when I laid on the radiation table.
- Making me cards, paintings, and quilts.
- Reading my CaringBridge posts so I didn't feel so alone on the journey.
- Texting me a mediation app, Bible verses, a word of encouragement, or just to say that you also hate that I am going through this.
- Bringing our family lemons, Korean pears, flowers, or a danish from Copenhagen Bakery.
- Letting my kids adopt your dog.
- Being a friend when you hardly knew me.
- Driving me to and from UCLA spa day.
- Bringing my mom to the hospital to be with me.
- Taking my kids to their practice and games.
- Coming to visit me.
- Inviting me for tea.
- Playing Lauren Daigle for me.

- Climbing Mt. Kilimanjaro with my name on a prayer flag.
- Staying with us: cooking meals, taking care of the kids, doing countless loads of laundry.
- Sending cold hard cash for me to get a mani-pedi, a treat, pay for medical bills, or whatever else our family needed.
- Taking a break from your busy day to call or text when you thought of me.
- Treating me to coffee, lunch, or dinner.
- Making me laugh and smile—even on the darkest days.
- Not being awkward around me because you didn't know what to say.
- Giving me a high five.
- Taking me to see Lauren Daigle in concert.
- Helping me find a wig that makes me feel beautiful.
- Sending my kids books, toys, and gifts to love on them.
- Seeing my beauty whether I am blonde, brunette, or bald.
- Telling me how amazing I look.
- Telling me that I'm your hero.
- Reminding me that "fso budet horosho."
- Coming to my home to pray for me.
- Believing for me when I couldn't.
- Going to work in the middle of the UC strike.
- Helping me to find my doctors at UCLA.

- Sharing your own cancer journey with me.
- Squeezing my hand during the hardest parts.
- Checking in with me by calling, FaceTiming, and Marco Poloing me.
- Shaving your head with me.
- Finding me a recliner and delivering it to me.
- Putting me on your prayer list.
- Taking me to the movies when I needed a couple hours to escape.
- Reminding me to go one more minute.
- Going for a walk with me.
- Going to doctor appointments with me.
- Showing me compassion and empathy.
- Giving me countless foot massages.
- Reminding me to be kind to myself.
- Talking me off the ledge.
- Playing handball with me and giving me a reason to get out of bed.
- Walking with me every step of the way and reminding me that God is greater than the highs and the lows.
- And all the things I failed to mention because there have just been too many to name. Thank you.

And to God...thank you for providing so many people to care for me and to be Your hands and feet to me. Thank you for healing me, hearing me, and redeeming even the darkest days.

Love,

Tanya

TO MY HALL-OF-FAMERS

NIKITA How can words even begin to thank you for all the ways you've shown up for me during this time? Thank you for sleeping on an uncomfortable hospital "bouch" (bed/couch) because you didn't want to leave me. And I'll never forget you kneeling by my recliner when I couldn't sleep on my side yet post-surgery and you just listened to me share all the things I was scared of, and you didn't try to fix it, you just held my hand and cried with me. Thank you for stepping up by cooking more and caring for our kids when I just didn't have the strength to.

Thank you for always seeing my beauty, before I lost my hair, when I had a mohawk, when I was bald, when I was wearing my wigs, and even when I had an awkward "permed" mullet after chemo. Thank you for reminding me that "fco budet horosho," even when you didn't know how it would be okay. For buying me my $1 filing cabinet...the best gift ever. For sticking by my side when I needed you most. And thank you for pointing me to Jesus and praying for me when I wasn't sure that I wanted anything to do with Him. I can't imagine anyone else I'd want by my side. You're my best buddy :-) and I could never have the words to describe my love and deep gratitude for you.

MY KIDS—HOPE, SOPHIA, & ZION You are the bravest humans I know. First, we told you that we were leaving behind our home, friends, and life in Seattle to head for California. Then, you started at a new school when you didn't know a soul and we had just moved into our rental three days before that. You became fast friends with our neighbors (and their dogs), and then you began to ask if we could stay after school to play because you had already made new friends. Just a few weeks later we told you that I had to have surgery to remove the cancer in my breast, and you didn't even know what cancer meant. A couple months after that I lost my hair and you had to answer your friends when they asked why I had long brown hair one day, and short blonde hair the next. And you tried church after church before we settled on Vintage because it was the first church you didn't complain about (and we happened to love it, too). You bravely met with Sheila to talk through your feelings, and you asked me tough questions and sometimes you cried with me. But through it all, you showed me your resilience and you've taught me what it means to persevere even when you don't know what is coming next. And most of all you showed me how to keep laughing and loving life, even when you're scared. I love you to the moon and back.

ALL THE GUYS WHO WERE THERE FOR NIKITA You were a God-send to Nikita (and me) because I knew that even though I couldn't care for him in the same way I normally would, God was caring for him through each of you. Thank you for being his companions during his darkest night of the soul. You were his life preservers. Thank you for being intentional with him by asking him to grab coffee, going on men's retreats with him, sending him encouraging texts, holding him accountable, taking him under your wing, and teaching him to surf. Your prayers for him sustained him, and your work outs together did more than strengthen his body. Thank you for stopping by, walking across the street, and calling him when you were thinking of him (even if he didn't call you back). In short, thank you for caring for my man, so that he was filled up to care for me.

LAUREN DAIGLE Thank for you singing songs that helped me put words to what I was feeling.

MOM I don't even want to consider what it would be like for me to get a call from one of my daughters saying that they had breast cancer. I can only imagine what was running through your head and your heart. Thank you for not freaking out, even if you were inside. I'm so thankful that God brought us back to SoCal to be closer to you. Thank you for buying me my first wig (something I never thought I'd say), coming to stay with us, watching my kids while I was in the hospital and going through treatment, folding our laundry, praying for us constantly, and just being with us in the darkness. Your presence brought us all peace. I love you so much.

TARA Thank you for your love and faithfulness not only for me, but for the kids and Nikita. Thank you for posting on CaringBridge and organizing the Meal Train so that we could share our needs with others. And thank you for coming to stay with us and spoiling us. You are a Tasmanian Devil-cooking-cleaning-laundry-folding-machine. (Steve, Justice, and Walker, thanks for loaning your wife and mom to us to help us through the toughest times). Love you all.

TODD & IRENE Thank you for caring for my kids and driving mom back and forth while I was in the hospital. Thank you for checking in on me. It was such a comfort knowing you were close. Todd, thank you for being steady and reminding me of what Dad would have said to me. Love you both.

THE DOCTOR FROM SWEDISH BREAST IMAGING I have no idea what your name is, but thank you for insisting on more images. I hate what you told me, but you started the process of saving my life. Thank you.

DR. DENNIS WOO You were the first person outside of our family that I told about my diagnosis. Thank for the compassion, calm, and understanding I could hear in your voice, for reminding me what Job said to God, for getting me in to see Dr. Chang, for checking in on me, and for being the perfect blend of doctor and friend.

ALL THOSE WHO CAME TO VISIT AND SERVED OUR FAMILY Your presence and care for me and my family, brought sunshine on the darkest days and reminded me that we weren't alone.

KARRIE & SHEILA It's hard to find a good counselor. I feel blessed to have found two. Thank you for caring for the hearts and souls of my family and me at different times in this journey. I would still be in the fetal position if it weren't for you two.

LIBERTY Thank you for being such a dear friend to me especially during this unspeakably difficult time. Thank you for inviting me into your community in LA, when I didn't have energy to build my own.

TREE, JEN, LINDS, & JULIE Thank you for consistently texting, calling, and praying for me throughout this journey. Even though you weren't close in proximity, you were very near.

KINDERGARTEN MOMS Thank you for not avoiding me because I was the new mom at school who had cancer. Thanks for your smiling faces, easy conversation, and our much needed Girls' Nights Out where I could laugh, eat delicious food, drink good wine, and not have to talk about cancer.

DR. CANALE Thank you for talking me off the ledge, reminding me to be kind to myself, listening to all my woes and fears, reassuring me, and giving me permission to be right where I am.

JAN I was so scared as I first sat in the waiting room of the UCLA REVLON Breast Center, but I instantly felt better once I walked through the door and saw you. We had only spoken on the phone, but when I asked, "Are you Jan?", you gave me a hug like you had known me your whole life. You reminded me of God's presence and anointing on my life.

DR. CHANG Even though my head was spinning from all the information you were throwing at me, I could tell that you were brilliant and professional, as well as compassionate and understanding. When I discovered that you had also faced breast cancer, I knew that I was in the right hands. I cannot thank you enough.

DR. DA LIO My personal Michaelangelo. Grazie for letting me cry in your office and for being so patient with me as you helped me process options for surgery. Thank you for making me laugh, giving such great life advice, and creating a masterpiece. Oh, and thank you for being the absolute best at what you do.

DR. OLEVSKY I have PTSD every time I have to come see you, but it's not because of you. It's just a reminder of the hell I've been through.

Thank you for caring for me uniquely, listening well, asking about Nikita and the kids, and obliterating any remaining cancer cells. If you were playing Space Invaders, you'd get the high score every time. Thank you for reminding me, "Fco budet horosho."

DR. MC CLOSKEY You are so good at what you do. Thank you for creating a peaceful space and a team that cares deeply about each patient coming for radiation therapy. There was no doubt in my mind that I was in the perfect place for my therapy. And yes, I will bring you monkey bread again. :)

PJ AND KELLY You are my 10:15 a.m. dream team. You guys are seriously the best. You helped make six weeks of radiation bearable.

You wipe tears, you bring laughter, you compliment my wigs, you're my personal DJ's. Thank you for fighting this battle with me.

HOLLY AT THE GILDED LILY Thank you for your heart to bring beauty and dignity to me and so many other women by sharing your artistic gift. Not only did you help to restore my breasts, you cared for my heart by listening well. Thank you for tattooing until it was just right.

ALL WHO SHARED THEIR CANCER JOURNEY WITH ME I'm so thankful for each of you coming alongside me by sending care packages, praying, walking with me, taking me to lunch, sharing your cancer journeys with me, showing me the ropes, crying with me, encouraging me, and reminding me that I'm not alone.

"THE BEST BARRINGTON AVE. CROWD" You became fast friends to our family. Thank you for not just smiling and waving, but taking time to cry with us, cheer us on, check in, bring meals and treats, and love us well. Thank you for being the most AMAZING neighbors we could have asked for.

MEL Thank you for capturing God's goodness and healing touch in my life through pictures. You are so much more than a photographer and I feel privileged to have had you join me on this journey.

JOY AND THE PUNCHLINE TEAM Thank you for coming alongside me during the roughest draft of this project and helping me to pull out the beauty. You and your team played a vital role by encouraging me, helping me craft my vision for this book and sharpening me as a writer. Joy, thank you for investing in me and getting behind this project. And thank you for inviting us into the pool that day with you and your mom. Your words and your perspective solidify why I wanted to write this book.

RACHAEL, JODI, LESLEE You are trail blazers. Thank you for seeing a need and filling it by creating The Unknown Authors Club (theunknownauthorsclub.com). Through the UAC and *The Life of An Unknown Author,* you built a platform for me and other unknown authors to stand on and be heard, which in turn grew my confidence and courage to publish *Covered: My Breast Cancer Story and Practical Insight for Yours.* Thank you for seeing the gold in the story that God has written for me and helping me to get this book into the hands of women who need it most. I am forever indebted to you.

GOD This wasn't the ministry I wanted or the story I would have written for myself, but I am thankful that You never left me (just like you promised). Your presence anchored me when I was certain the waves would swallow me. I will never be able to express the depths of my gratitude to You for healing me and giving me hope, even in my darkest hour. You deserve all the glory.

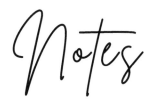

Notes

PREFACE

1. *The Problem of Pain*, C.S. Lewis. Revised ed. 2015, HarperOne.

CHAPTER 3

1. Psalm 29:10-11 The Holy Bible, New International Version

CHAPTER 4

1. Job 2:10 The Holy Bible, New Living Translation

CHAPTER 6

1. Lauren Daigle, "Rescue," Album: *Look Up Child*. Songwriters: Jason David Ingram / Lauren Daigle / Paul Brendon Mabury

CHAPTER 7

1. Jeremiah 29:11 The Holy Bible, New International Version
2. Hebrews 12:2 The Holy Bible, New Living Translation
3. Philippians 4:7 The Holy Bible, New International Version
4. Deuteronomy 11:8,18 The Holy Bible, New International Version

CHAPTER 8

1. John 11:1-44 The Holy Bible, New International Version
2. 1 Corinthians 13 The Holy Bible, New International Version
3. Psalm 23: 2, 4 The Holy Bible, New International Version

CHAPTER 9

1. Mark 2:1-12 The Holy Bible, New International Version
2. CaringBridge: caringbridge.com
3. Meal Train: mealtrain.com
4. Marco Polo application: Apple Store
5. *On Grief and Grieving: Finding the Meaning of Grief Through the Five Stages of Loss*, Elisabeth Kubler-Ross, David Kessler, Maria Shriver. Copyright 2005, 2014
6. *What About Bob?*, movie, 1991, directed by Frank Oz
7. "The Effect of a Christian-Based Support Group on the Emotional Health of Cancer Survivors and Caregivers", https://jnccn.org/view/journals/jnccn/19/3.5/article-pHSR21-056.xml HSR21-056
8. *Don't Waste Your Cancer* by John Piper 2011 by Desiring God Foundation
9. *It's Not Fair: Learning to Love the Life You Didn't Choose* by Melanie Dale, 2016 by Zondervan
10. *Pretty Sick: The Beauty Guid for Women with Cancer* by Caitlin M. Kiernan 2017, Grand Central Life & Style
11. *Walking with God Through Pain and Suffering* by Timothy Keller 2013, Penguin Books

CHAPTER 11

1. *The 7 Habits of Highly Effective People* by Stephen R. Covey 1999, 2004, 2020, Simon & Schuster
2. *The Tonight Show Starring Jimmy Fallon*, TV show, NBC
3. *EuroVision Song Contest: The Story of Fire Saga*, movie, 2020, Produced by Savan Kotecha

4. *Gilmore Girls,* TV show, 2000, created by Amy Sherman-Palladino
5. SoulSpace application found on the Apple Store

CHAPTER 13
1. Ecclesiastes 3:1 The Holy Bible, New International Version
2. Psalm 46:5 The Holy Bible, New International Version

CHAPTER 16
1. Isaiah 34:1-4 The Holy Bible, New International Version
2. Psalm 91:4 The Holy Bible, New International Version

CHAPTER 18
1. Joshua 1:1-9 The Holy Bible, New International Version

CHAPTER 19
1. Matthew 6:26-27 The Holy Bible, New International Version

CHAPTER 20
1. James 1:2-4 The Holy Bible, New International Version

CHAPTER 22
1. Exodus 17 The Holy Bible, New International Version

CHAPTER 25
1. *Pretty Sick: The Beauty Guid for Women with Cancer* by Caitlin M. Kiernan, 2017, Grand Central Life & Style

CHAPTER 27
1. *My Cancer Journey,* by Dr. Pam Evans, Polly Noble, and Nicholas Hull-Malham

2. *Forks Over Knives,* documentary, 2011, Netflix
3. *The Wellness Remodel* by Christina Anstead and Cara Clark
4. *Feeding You Lies: How to Unravel the Food Industry's Playbook and Reclaim Your Health* by Vani Hari 2020 Hay House Inc.
5. *Food Babe Kitchen: More than 100 Delicious Real Food Recipes to Change Your Body and Your Life* by Vani Hari 2020 Hay House Inc.
6. *The Pegan Diet: 21 Practical Principles for Reclaiming Your Health in a Nutritionally Confusing World* by Dr. Mark Hyman MD, 2021, Little, Brown Spark
7. *Food: What the Heck Should I Cook?* by Dr. Mark Hyman MD, 2019, Little, Brown Spark

CHAPTER 28
1. Psalm 139:14 The Holy Bible, New International Version

CHAPTER 30
1. "Kintsugi", *Magnolia Journal*, Fall 2019

CHAPTER 31
1. 2 Corinthians 5:17 The Holy Bible, New International Version
2. Brené Brown on Empathy, www.youtube.com/watch?v=1Evwgu369Jw
3. Psalm 46:5 The Holy Bible, New International Version

ABOUT TANYA MOTORIN

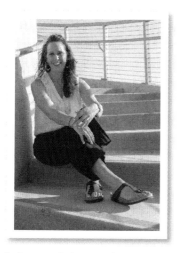

TANYA MOTORIN is a first-time author who always thought she had a book in her, but didn't know what to write about. When she was diagnosed with breast cancer in July 2018, she knew her first book would be about her breast cancer journey. As a breast cancer survivor, her hope is that through vulnerability and sharing her personal experience, she will encourage and help other women feel known, cared for, and resourced as they walk through their own journeys with breast cancer. Tanya has been on staff full-time with Athletes in Action, an international Christian sport ministry, since 2002. She and her husband are currently serving the athletic community at UCLA and the LA coastline. She loves spending time writing, creating, organizing, cooking, buying more than she needs at Target, and getting some self-care by going on a hike or a long walk. Tanya also loves spending time with friends and family, traveling, going to the beach, camping, laughing hard, and watching a good movie. She and her husband, Nikita, live in Mar Vista, California with their daughters, Hope and Sophia, their son, Zion, and their Chiweenie, Daisy.